T0220349

Handbook of Physician Mental Health

This definitive textbook on Practitioner Health mixes academic rigour with practitioner and patient experiences. The book covers all aspects of care relevant to any regulated health professional, focusing on the care of doctors and nurses with mental illness. The book builds on themes introduced in the award-winning publication *Beneath the White Coat: Doctors, Their Minds and Mental Health* from the same author. It provides an invaluable 'how to manage' companion to supplement and enhance the broader issues relating to doctors and mental illness addressed in that first book.

Drawing together 15 years of expertise in caring for more than 30,000 doctors with mental illness, the book is relevant to any health professional working in clinical practice and will be essential reading for those who regulate, appraise, train and support health practitioners across various disciplines.

Handbook of Physician Mental Health

Professor Dame Clare Gerada
Founder of NHS Practitioner Health
Past President, Royal College of General Practitioners
UK

With contributions from
Dr Sarinda Wijetunge
Doctors in Distress
UK

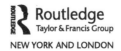

Routledge
Taylor & Francis Group

NEW YORK AND LONDON

Designed cover image: Shutterstock

First edition published 2025
by Routledge
605 Third Ave., 21st Floor, New York, NY 10158

and by Routledge
4 Park Square, Milton Park, Abingdon, Oxon, OX14 4RN

Routledge is an imprint of Taylor & Francis Group, LLC

© 2025 Clare Gerada

ISBN: 978-1-032-48937-7 (hbk)
ISBN: 978-1-032-47986-6 (pbk)
ISBN: 978-1-003-39150-0 (ebk)

DOI: 10.1201/9781003391500

Typeset in Minion Pro
by KnowledgeWorks Global Ltd.

Contents

Introduction, acknowledgements and about the author and contributors

We thank Routledge Publishers for publishing this handbook. It was written by Clare (primary author, a general practitioner [GP] working with mentally ill doctors for two decades) with support from Sarinda (a junior doctor with live experience of mental ill health). Both of us bring our own and collective knowledge to this book. Others, particularly clinicians at Practitioner Health, have also contributed to this book in different ways, and we thank them.

Let us introduce the primary author and contributor.

I am Clare Gerada, the principal author of this book, and this is my story.

My choice to be a doctor was, as for many, influenced by a close family member. My late father, a GP, ran a single-handed practice in East England for years. Like many doctors in the 1960s, he came as an immigrant to work in the newly formed but struggling National Health Service. For several years, my father's surgery was also our family home. Our living room doubled up as the patient's waiting room, meaning that during the day, when not at school, all five children were forced to tip-toe quietly upstairs. Our dining room doubled as his consulting room; the dining table was covered with the old Lloyd George patient records. My earliest memories were peering over the upstairs balcony and seeing strangers below, mainly women and small children. I was intrigued by their presence and the noises they made as they waited to see my father. Later, he would take me on home visits – where I would wait excitedly in the car for him to return from the visit and tell me what he saw. He taught me that to be a good GP, one had to listen to patients, be part of their community and provide continuity of care. My father was well-loved and a pillar of the local community, and wherever I went, home, school, church or the local market, patients entered my world daily.

Given my idealisation of my father, it is no coincidence that I tried to emulate him and make him proud of me. I went to medical school and qualified as a doctor years later, eventually becoming a GP. My surgery does not so much double up as my sitting room but is nevertheless within metres of my home, and my professional and personal lives are intertwined.

While my reasons for entering medicine might seem healthy, they nevertheless pre-disposed me to a career of constantly aspiring to be better, needing to prove myself and never being satisfied by my achievements. For others, the reason they chose to become doctors might be related to early traumas – the classic Wounded Healer, which will be touched on later.

Here is Sarinda's story:

My parents were immigrants from Sri Lanka. My father left to be educated in the UK at a young age, and my mother was a medical student seeking to continue her studies away from the civil war. As with many who leave so much behind, they dealt with their failed ambitions by vicariously promoting mine. They instilled in me the need to work hard, succeed and do better than my peers. They spent consid-erable money on my education, a good investment on paper as I excelled academi-cally in music and sport and was envied as an 'all-rounder'. Behind this success was what I kept hidden. I was one of only a few children in the school who were non-White. I experienced abuse, taunting and what is now called a 'hate crime'. The racism reached its climax when I entered the 6th form. Boys threw coins at me each morning as an advanced 'payment' for their racist comments. These were vile words where teachers feigned deafness. One day, I returned home from school with a broken arm. My response was to work harder, to 'show them all'. By working, I could distract myself and seek revenge for my success over theirs. I wanted to study medicine for my interest in the sciences, but I now know that my choice was made not just to fix me but to fix others who felt as I did.

As I entered medical school, I was excited and eager to learn. However, my early enthusiasm quickly waned by the third year as I struggled to keep up with the workload and the pressure. I felt like an 'imposter' and was only there because of my parent's expectations. I was constantly anxious and overwhelmed and fell into a pattern of overworking to compensate for my insecurities.

At the same time, I began to see the darker side of medicine. I saw doctors who were dismissive and rude to their patients, who seemed to care more about their egos than the well-being of the people they were supposed to be helping. I saw the impact of a system that valued costs over people, where patients were treated like commodities and doctors were pushed to their limits by the job's demands.

All of this started to take a toll on my mental health. I became increasingly isolated and depressed, and I struggled to find anyone to talk to who could understand what I was going through. My parents, who had invested so much in my education, couldn't grasp the challenges I faced. I felt I was drowning and didn't know how to seek help.

It took a long time for me to realise that I wasn't alone and that others had gone through similar struggles. I started to connect with other health professionals who shared their stories of burnout, anxiety and depression. I began to see that my strug-gles were not a sign of weakness but a reflection of a broken system that needed fixing.

Through it all, I learned the importance of self-care and the need to prioritise my well-being. I sought help from a physician's health service and saw a psychiatrist who persuaded me to take a year off. Therapy and antidepressants helped my recovery, and I restarted my training. I made a new group of friends to join for the final year. I thrived, and I learned to love again. I was determined to be as good a doctor no matter what, one who was compassionate and caring. I passed the medical school, obtaining a distinction, to my disbelief.

During the pandemic, I thrived and felt needed and valuable, but as with many doctors working during this time, I felt overwhelmed by my encounters with death. So much death. Handovers turned into running down a list of who would die that night. I grew to resent medicine once more in Foundation Year 2. I wouldn't say I enjoyed coming to work.

I burst into tears at an accident and emergency morning handover and was surrounded by the kind, loving arms of the department's consultants. There was plenty of compassion for me as I bawled my eyes out. People are wonderful. I wished the system cared for its staff like that. I wanted the system to allow staff time and space to care for each other like that. There seemed never to be time.

I took time off, only a few weeks. I returned to child and adolescent mental health. This was where I found my love for psychiatry and mental health. I know that some days, I wore the mask of a cheerful joker at work, whose energy was boundless and carried me through the day, but other days, I felt I could just 'be' and enjoy living. This was merely temporary. I had planned to end my life following a work party I had organised. It did not go according to plan, and I was admitted to a mental health unit for two weeks. I sought help from Practitioner Health. I went through cognitive behavioural therapy coaching and have been reading the great literary works of wise men and women. I was never alone. I am human. No one is unbreakable.

I have learned much through a dark experience of training in medicine, and as a patient in an overburdened mental health system, what is truly up to me and within my control: My power of choice. I put so much desire and attachment into what should be fair and just for myself and others that whatever at the time seemed an injustice caused me to fall into anger, sadness and despair. Working to prevent what happened to me from happening to others, even simply trying, is undoubtedly in my power and aligns with my values. I have learned to stick to my principles and am now in the best place of my life. In sum, I am grateful for all that medicine has shown me: It takes courage and discipline to use your time and space wisely for the best interests of yourself and others.

The book is aimed at any health professional working in a caring or supervisory, mentoring or pastoral role with another health professional. It is mainly for those in UK practice who care for fellow healthcare professionals as patients/mentees/ supervisees. Issues discussed predominantly relate to medical doctors but are inevitably familiar to any health practitioner within a regulatory framework. It aims to be a '*how to do*' (and '*what not to do*') in managing doctors with mental illness. Still, it also touches on broader socio-political issues that might not be in the treating practitioner's gift to change but are essential to understanding their impact on clinicians' mental health. These include the culture and working environment, training and workforce issues and how organisations and systems in which the practitioner works can be both protective, though currently, and sadly are, more often, harmful.

Doctors do not suffer from different mental illnesses from their patients. Where they do vary in how (more often, how not) they present for care, the potential impact of their illness on their patients, how this might need to be addressed and where necessary, involving their regulatory or employing or training body. Other differences relate to how others perceive illness in health professionals and how denial of vulnerability in the sick doctor and those treating the ill doctor might affect future management. For doctors, mental illness is often their shameful secret, hidden from sight. This means many depressed and anxious doctors are denied help (usually through their reluctance to seek it). Hopefully, this handbook will contribute to doctors being treated humanely and skilled wherever they might present.

The term 'health professional' indicates any individual working in a regulated system within the health system. The term doctor defines any individual with medical (doctor) training.

Unless otherwise stated, all vignettes are fictitious, though they are based on thousands of doctors presenting for care at Practitioner Health.

Setting the scene

The genesis of this book stems from the NHS Practitioner Health (PH), a mental health service initially set up for doctors and dentists, but which since 2020 has been available to all regulated health professionals working in Scotland and England who face barriers accessing confidential mental health care. As of 2024, the service sees around 6,500 patients per year. This book stems from the learning accumulated over the last 15 years and from a competency framework developed by the service.

Beneath the White Coat: Doctors, Their Minds and Mental Illness,[1] written by one of the authors (CG), the former head of NHS PH, should be read alongside this handbook. *Beneath the White Coat* provides a contextual overview of the incidence, prevalence, aetiology and nature of mental illness among doctors.

As this book will discuss, the literature shows that:[2]

- Mental illness is common among doctors.

- Suicide rates are between two and four times those of other professional groups. General practitioners (GPs), psychiatrists, doctors trained overseas and women are especially at risk.

- Stigma and prejudice exacerbate mental health conditions.

- Patient complaints are a significant factor in leading to suicide among doctors.

Treating fellow health professionals can be challenging as several barriers prevent them from seeking appropriate help.

These include the following:

- Lack of knowledge about where to seek help, especially for junior doctors who frequently move around different areas for training or newly arrived international medical graduates.

- Personality factors contribute to the denial of vulnerability. These include factors such as obsessiveness, martyrdom and competitiveness.

- Concerns about professional implications (i.e., regulator involvement, detriment to career progression and the impact of having time off sick).

- Difficulties of disclosure are linked to stigma, prejudice, shame and fear of taking on the 'patient role'.

Doctors are at increased risk of mental illness due to factors including:

- **Professionalism:** Never leaving a job undone

- **Job:** Emotionally and physically exhausting

- **System:** Culture of shame, blame and name

PRACTITIONER HEALTH

Many barriers preventing doctors from seeking timely care came to light following the death of a young psychiatrist, Daksha Emson, in October 2000. Daksha was a psychiatrist with bipolar affective disorder. She developed a psychotic depression postpartum, which led to her killing herself and her baby daughter, Freya. The Department of Health established an independent Inquiry into the tragedy. More will be said about Daksha later in this handbook.

The Inquiry highlighted that the issues contributing most to the outcome were as follows:

- The stigma of mental illness

- The difficulties of simultaneously being a doctor and a patient

- Inadequacies in perinatal mental health services

- Being a child of a parent with mental illness

- Inadequacies in NHS occupational health services

One of the recommendations from the Inquiry was to produce a protocol for doctor-to-doctor consultations and to look at the nature and structure of services for doctors with physical or psychological illnesses. In 2006–2007, the London Deanery and Royal College of Psychiatrists formed an expert working group assisted by the National Clinical Assessment Service (NCAS) to develop proposals for a Practitioner Health Programme (PHP). In 2007, the White Paper *Trust, Assurance and Safety: The Regulation of Health Professionals in the 21st Century* recognised that the complexity of modern clinical practice was placing enormous pressure on health professionals and that more could be done to support them. Subsequently, the Department of Health tasked NCAS with overseeing the commissioning and implementation of a prototype PHP.

PHP, as it was then called, later changing its name to NHS PH, was founded in response. It was recognised at the time that whilst every clinician should be aware of the issues facing a sick health professional, there was a particular skill set in actively treating and supporting them. PHP opened its doors in 2008 as a confidential, self-referral service for doctors and dentists in London to access help for their mental health and addiction problems.

In 2017, NHS England commissioned a service for all GPs across England in response to the increasing pressures and poor attrition rates in the speciality. In early 2019, PHP became available to all doctors and dentists working in the English NHS, with Scotland being added a year later; it then changed its name to Practitioner Health (PH), which we shall use from now onwards. As a result of the pandemic and from 2020, all health staff (with some eligibility criteria) can now access the service.

The service was the first of its kind in the UK (nationally funded, free at the point of use) and has become one of the world's most extensive physician health services at the time of writing. It provides interventions typically found in a standard outpatient mental health department, with the addition of inpatient treatment for addiction. Clinicians can prescribe medicines and various psychological interventions, including group, remote, face-to-face and web-based therapy.

PH exemplifies the truism '*if you build it, they will come*'. The doors to the service were opened in September 2008, and within minutes, the first patient made contact. Nearly two decades later, more than 30,000 have sought help.

Over the years, around 80% of the patients presenting to the service suffer from mental health problems, 10% have a substance misuse problem, and the rest have a mix of other diagnoses. Of those with mental health problems, around 80% have anxiety, depression, obsessive–compulsive disorder or adjustment disorder; the remaining 20% have serious mental health problems, mostly eating disorders or bipolar affective disorder, and a few have a personality disorder or psychosis. For substance misuse, around 75% are related to predominantly alcohol misuse, 10% to drug use and the remainder to behavioural addictions or mixed drug and alcohol.

The nature and type of mental illnesses have not changed significantly since the service started accepting patients for treatment in 2008.

PH stands out for its high-quality care due to its specialist expertise in caring for doctors and management with tailored, holistic support for their needs. The clinicians who work with PH are attuned to the doctor's illness in a way that allows for safer treatment and streamlined management from first consultation to discharge. At the root of the service is an in-depth understanding of the complexities of this patient group. The service was rated as outstanding by the Care Quality Commission in 2018.

COMPETENCES

This book hopes to equip the reader with the following:

Clinical

- A good understanding and implementation of self-care and competence in advising practitioner–patients on self-care

- Ability to provide first-contact care and assessments for practitioner–patients

- Providing continuing care and signposting to a range of clinical interventions such as cognitive behavioural therapy, group therapy and other treatments as appropriate

- Management of mental health and addiction problems as far as individual expertise allows

Education and liaison

- Providing advice and liaison to other practitioners through remote or face-to-face contact to manage those problems/conditions within their expertise

- Providing support and training to other health practitioners in areas related to the prevention, identification and brief intervention of mental health/addiction problems in health professionals, as well as self-care and well-being

- Liaising with other practitioners involved in the care of practitioner–patients

Other

- Supporting a return-to-work programme

- Understanding the regulatory framework

PRACTITIONER HEALTH (UK) *VERSUS* PHYSICIAN HEALTH (NORTH AMERICA)

Early in this handbook, it is worth laying out the differences and similarities between NHS PH and other physician health programmes, especially those in North America. Physician (doctor) only services addressing doctors' mental health have operated since the 1970s. The earliest ones were established in North America, with doctors volunteering to help colleagues with mental health and substance misuse problems. They were set up in response to calls from the American health authorities, alarmed by the risks posed to physicians with addiction and psychiatric illness and the high number of physician suicides in those who had experienced revocation of their licence to practise (equivalent to erasure in the UK).

Since then, physician health programmes have developed mainly across North America and Canada, though others are in different parts of the world. These programmes are more akin to a probation service – where the addicted health professional is mandated as part of the engagement programme to submit themselves to formal testing for the use of drugs/alcohol, supervision, regular assessment, information gathering and reports to the doctor's employer and regulator.

North American physician health programmes (PHP) do not provide treatment per se. Instead, they provide evaluation and diagnosis, develop a contract detailing treatment or monitoring, coordinate and facilitate formal treatment through accredited providers and ongoing professional support and carry out regular monitoring through random visits to places of work and regular screenings for alcohol and drugs, typically for five years.

American physician health services act as an intermediary between the doctor, the regulator, or their employer, ensuring that the doctor receives and adheres to

Table 1.1 Comparison between the American and UK physician health programmes

	USA PHP based 904 doctors enrolled into 16 PHPs	NHS Practitioner Health based on 10 years
Referrals	Self-referral is unusual	100% self-referrals
Assessment	Typically 2–5 days multidisciplinary evaluation	90-minute assessment by PH clinician
Multidisciplinary team (MDT)	MDT involved in care planning, assessing risk and any other issues based on the assessment	MDT involved in care planning, assessing risk and any other issues based on the assessment
Contract	Stipulating abstinence, sharing of information, adhering to treatment, requirements to work under supervision, testing	None
Treatment	Mandated pathway involving approved providers	Patients given choice of treatment options
Residential Rehab	30–90 days of residential treatment or community-based treatment. Around 70% doctors have residential care	6 weeks of other community-based treatment or residential treatment. Around 25% have residential care
Testing	Intensive random, unannounced, drug and alcohol testing for 20 drugs or more, testing weekly or twice weekly at start (e.g., first 2 years), then less after (20 times per year) for around 5 years. 75% of all urine samples were supervised	Only tested if clinically indicated – typically at the start of treatment. No observed urine testing. Testing is urine (70%) blood (10%), hair (20%)
Work	Workplace monitoring	Cannot stipulate any monitoring
Confidentiality	Requirement for information sharing	MoU with GMC with respect to needing to breach confidentiality
Supervision/ Follow up	Must meet, with frequency determined by case manager	As necessary based on each individual case
12 Steps	Required	Recommended
Other treatment	Must attend individual and group work as required by contract	As determined by individual care planning. All voluntary
Funding	Self-funded	NHS
Abstinence based	Uniformly abstinent based	Allows some controlled drinking
Adjunctive medication	Unusual, but prescribed as needed. For example, 1 out of 904 doctors were placed on methadone for opiate-dependence	Unusual, but prescribed as needed. 2 out of 400 placed on buprenorphine for opiate-dependence

recommended treatment. They usually work directly with referring professional societies, medical centres, colleagues and families to assess and intervene with affected doctors to convince them of the need for professional long-term care. Another common feature of American PHPs is the signed contract between the PHP and the physician participant, specifying the elements of care and monitoring, the reporting practices and potential consequences for noncompliance. They also strongly recommend (essentially mandating) abstinence-oriented treatment and admission to residential programmes. There is also an expectation that any recurrence of drug/alcohol use has to be disclosed and forms part of a decision for the clinician's fitness to practise. Whilst subsidised, physician health services in North America are nevertheless self- (or insurance-funded), with costs for a doctor attending rising to hundreds of thousands of dollars over their involvement. In recent years, these programmes have drawn criticism as being coercive, expensive and lacking transparency. Nevertheless, their outcomes are good, with only around 20% of doctors entering the programme testing positive during the five years and more than 70% continuing to work.[3]

Unlike their North American counterparts, NHS PH is not part of a regulatory or disciplinary process. The equivalent of North American PH in the UK would be a doctor under regulatory (General Medical/Dental Council) conditions to undertake supervision, treatment, testing and monitoring through their accredited psychiatrists. PH is not affiliated with, nor does it have any reporting requirements to, the doctor's employer, regulator, or any other body or individual. Other than in exceptional circumstances, it does not breach confidentiality, and patients are not mandated to follow any treatment or monitoring regime (though they are strongly encouraged to do so). PH only monitors adherence if it adds to the patient's care, not as part of any performance, disciplinary or regulatory requirement. This does not mean that PH is not obligated to disclose to the doctor's employer or regulator if there are concerns that their behaviour or mental illness might be impacting their fitness to practise, only that monitoring adherence to strict treatment regimens is not part of PH's remit.

2

The Wounded Healer

This handbook has already used the idea of the 'Wounded Healer'. It is a term used for any caring professional who has personal experience of mental (or physical) injury, trauma or challenges and uses this experience to care for others. These personal experiences can provide the carer with unique insights, empathy and understanding when working with those dealing with similar issues. Drawing from their own experiences and growth, the Wounded Healer may be better equipped to provide support, guidance and healing to others. Experience helps to channel personal suffering for the betterment of others.

Suffering is part of the human experience, and everyone carries psychological, emotional, physical and even spiritual traumas from the past. Sigmund Freud, the founder of psychoanalysis, suggested that we are all prone to repeat past traumas, which forms the basis of much psychoanalytic practice. Choosing a medical career provides the theatre for playing out the wounded, unresolved part of one's past. It is not uncommon for a doctor to select a speciality based on their experience. For example, becoming a paediatrician might be related to having suffered from illness during childhood or being an addiction specialist due to parental alcoholism. These unconscious motives can be a driving force for compassion and commitment but also a foreshadowing of mental illness if not understood and kept in check, primarily through supervision or facilitated reflective practice. A medical career can act as a defence against feelings of anxiety or impotence resulting from the experience of illness or death in family members. A pattern might be established where the doctor is so invested in an unconscious and unrealistic desire to *heal their wounds*, sublimated through caring for others, that they risk becoming overly involved with patients, transgressing professional boundaries, or developing burnout, anxiety or depression.

The construct of the '**Wounded Healer**' is part of Greek mythology. Hercules accidentally wounded the immortal demigod Chiron with a poisoned arrow; the wound never healed and caused him immense pain. Chiron chose to transform his suffering into helping others until he was eventually able to die by exchanging his life for Prometheus and, through death, becoming free from pain. Chiron was a kind, gentle man; he was a teacher, and before his death, he gave himself

DOI: 10.1201/9781003391500-2

tirelessly to others and used his gift to reduce suffering in his fellow man. The myth of Chiron is the basis of the modern concept of the Wounded Healer: The doctor, therapist or other professional who gives to others.

The Swiss psychiatrist Carl Jung explored the Wounded Healer concept as an archetypal psychological pattern. He emphasised that individuals who confront and integrate their psychological wounds can develop a greater empathy and emotional understanding. This process allows them to navigate their challenges and extend a healing presence to those in need.

The Wounded Healer is a resonant archetype with profound significance across cultures, history and psychological understanding. It symbolises a transformative journey from personal pain to healing and ultimately assisting others on their paths to recovery. This concept encapsulates that those who have experienced and overcome their wounds, challenges and struggles can offer unique healing and empathy to others undergoing similar trials.

At its core, it underscores the interconnectedness of human experiences. It acknowledges that through our struggles and vulnerabilities, we gain an empathetic insight into the pain of others. This understanding is the foundation for a healing relationship that transcends clinical knowledge and delves into genuine connection.

Modern society has seen the Wounded Healer archetype take shape in various fields, from counselling and therapy to addiction recovery. Personal experience of mental illness, particularly alcohol or drug misuse, has driven the recovery movement, with organisations such as the British Doctors & Dentists Group (BDDG) set up by health professionals with an addiction drawn from the medical and dental profession. Individuals who have emerged from personal struggles with mental health, addiction, trauma or other challenges often find themselves uniquely equipped to guide others through similar difficulties. Their lived experiences foster a deep sense of empathy and provide a tangible source of hope, proving that healing is possible.

Ultimately, the Wounded Healer archetype invites individuals to view their wounds as sources of strength rather than shame. It reminds us that our struggles are not in vain; they can be transformed into wellsprings of wisdom, compassion and empowerment. By embracing our vulnerabilities and working through challenges, we can transcend our pain and actively contribute to the healing of others. The concept of the Wounded Healer also reminds us that healing is not a solitary endeavour but a shared journey. It encourages us to be open to giving and receiving support, highlighting the potential for positive transformation that arises when one channels pain into purpose.

The Wounded Healer concept has deep roots in various cultural and therapeutic traditions. It acknowledges that carers, like anyone else, can face their life challenges, including experiences of trauma, mental health issues, addiction or other personal difficulties. These experiences can be seen as a source of vulnerability and a potential strength in the therapeutic relationship.

Key points when exploring the concept of the Wounded Healer include:

1. **Empathy and understanding:** A health professional who has overcome their wounds may have a heightened sense of empathy and understanding for their patients. This can create a strong rapport and trust in the therapeutic relationship, as patients often feel more comfortable opening up to someone who has 'been there'.

2. **Shared experience:** Personal experiences can provide a sense of shared experience and connection. Patients may be more inclined to listen to someone who has faced similar challenges and emerged from them, as they may view the therapist as a role model for recovery and growth.

3. **Personal growth:** The Wounded Healer archetype emphasises that health professionals are not infallible. They are constantly evolving as individuals. Their healing journey can contribute to their ongoing personal and professional development.

4. **Boundaries and self-care:** While personal experiences can be valuable, health professionals must ensure that their wounds do not interfere with their ability to provide practical, unbiased patient care.

5. **Supervision and support:** Wounded Healers often seek supervision and support to ensure their personal experiences do not negatively impact their practice. This helps maintain professional ethics and standards.

6. **Integration of personal experience:** Effective Wounded Healers are skilled at integrating their personal experiences into their therapeutic approach to benefit patients without making the therapy about their journey.

Many of these issues will be expanded upon later in this handbook.

3

Doctors and mental illness

What follows is a brief overview of the mental disorders seen among doctors.

BURNOUT

Maria, a consultant physician, burst through the cubicle curtains and banged straight into the notes trolley hip-first. 'Why are we still using piles of paper'? she barked, 'for goodness' sake!' She felt irritated and sadly disinterested in what faced her that day. She had seen it all before, and 'why are they bothering me?' The junior doctor began to present the patient to her yet, sensing his consultant's irritation, stumbled over his words. 'Quickly'! she said, 'I have a clinic in an hour'. She snatched the notes from the junior, scolding him for wasting her time by not prepping the case. After she slammed the notes back onto the trolley, she looked up; tears fell down his reddened face. The young man turned slowly and walked out of the cubicle, and she heard the ward door close behind him. She buried her head in her hands. 'I don't even know his name...'.

Burnout is not a mental illness, though some of its features can be indistinguishable from depression or anxiety. The World Health Organisation (WHO) International Classification of Diseases (ICD) recognises burnout as an occupational rather than a medical condition. The recent ICD-11 (2019) describes burnout as '*resulting from chronic workplace stress that has not been successfully managed*'. Burnout and depression can have similar symptoms, such as hopelessness, low self-esteem and sleep disturbance. However, burnout is a distinct condition related explicitly to long-term job stress and a lack of personal accomplishment. It shares many features with depression and anxiety, and they often coexist.

Whilst linked, **stress** and burnout are not the same. Stress refers to temporary adaptation (with positive and negative connotations) accompanied by physical and mental symptoms ('*flight fight responses*'). Stress can have positive aspects, driving individuals to be more alert and focused on their work. In contrast, burnout is the final stage in a breakdown of the person's ability to adapt, which results

 DOI: 10.1201/9781003391500-3

from the long-term imbalance between demands and resources. It occurs when it is impossible to achieve anymore; inadequate resources or lack of autonomy make it impossible to accomplish work goals, and frustration erodes the spirit. Burnout can be a precursor to mental illness.

Surveys over the last five decades have consistently shown that around a third of doctors are suffering from burnout at any one time, regardless of the speciality or health system in which they work. It is fair to say that almost all doctors presenting to care for mental health issues have an element of burnout, and all those in a caring profession will suffer from burnout at some point in their careers. It is impossible not to. What is essential is to recognise when one is becoming disillusioned, unempathetic and disengaging with caring for others.

Burnout can be summarised in three dimensions:[4]

- **Chronic exhaustion:** Physically, emotionally and mentally
- **Depersonalisation:** A disengagement from self, others and the job
- **Lack of personal efficacy:** A diminished sense of accomplishment

While diagnostic tools are used in research to help establish prevalence rates of burnout in clinical practice, assessing the level, that is, the numerical severity of symptoms, is often not helpful. What is useful is acknowledging the demoralisation, exhaustion and lack of interest in the job.

Individuals might describe a host of subjective experiences, such as:

'I just don't care about this anymore'.

'What is the point of doing this when I make no difference'?

'I am failing to be a good doctor'.

'I'm not getting enough sleep; I can't stand work any longer'.

'I don't feel anything, only numbness'.

The causes of burnout are like those of depression and anxiety, though work-related factors play a more significant part in the pathogenesis of their illness.

The consequences of burnout can be serious, which can negatively impact both the individual experiencing it and the quality of care they provide. Some doctors may become disengaged, while others may become detached and isolated. Still, others may try to compensate by working harder and taking on an excessive sense of responsibility, leading to feelings of anxiety and depression. Unaddressed burnout can also increase the risk of substance misuse, depression, anxiety and suicide.

Table 3.1 Causes of burnout	
Summary of the causes of burnout	
Work related	Having little or no control over work
	Lack of recognition or reward for good work
	Unclear or overly demanding job expectations
	Doing work that is monotonous or unchallenging
	Working in a chaotic or high-pressure environment
Lifestyle	Poor sleep
	Working too much, without enough time for socialising or relaxing
	Lack of close, supportive relationships
	Taking on too many responsibilities, without enough help from others
Personality traits	*Perfectionistic tendencies*: Nothing is ever good enough
	Pessimism
	The need to be in control
	Reluctance to delegate to others
	High-achieving, competitive personality
Socio-political	Societies' unrealistic expectations of what doctors can do with medicine, leading to doctors being the container for fear, anxiety and disappointment
	Funding pressures can make it impossible to achieve the care needed

COMPASSION FATIGUE

Michael, a general practitioner (GP), had always prided himself on his ability to provide high-quality care to his patients. Over time, however, he noticed changes in himself, impacting his ability to maintain his usual level of empathy and engagement with his patients. One day, he was overwhelmed by the sheer volume of those needing his attention. He had back-to-back appointments, each with patients bringing their concerns and needs. As the day wore on, Michael felt a growing sense of fatigue and emotional heaviness. He started to experience a sense of detachment and found it increasingly difficult to connect with his patients on an emotional level. The emotional toll of his work began to weigh heavily on him, and he started to question his effectiveness as a doctor. He felt guilty for not being able to give each patient the attention and care they deserved.

Compassion fatigue is the loss of satisfaction from doing one's job well or job-related distress that outweighs job satisfaction. It can affect anyone working with patients in a healthcare environment, with doctors particularly vulnerable. Many factors can increase the risk of compassion fatigue, including non-supportive work settings, high caseloads and insufficient resources. Compassion fatigue can be due to personal, team and organisational factors, often a combination of all three. There is evidence that compassion fatigue can negatively impact a care provider's performance, morale and staff retention.[5] Below are features associated with compassion fatigue:

- Becoming pessimistic (thinking negative thoughts) or cynical.

- Becoming overly irritable or quick to anger.

- Withdrawal from social connections. This can become obvious in neglected friendships or relationships.

Compassion fatigue and burnout share some similarities but are not the same. Compassion fatigue refers to the emotional and physical exhaustion that healthcare professionals may experience because of prolonged exposure to the suffering and trauma of their patients. It is often characterised by a decreased ability to empathise and connect with patients, feelings of emotional numbness or detachment and a sense of being overwhelmed by the job demands. On the other hand, burnout is a more general term that refers to chronic physical and emotional exhaustion caused by prolonged and excessive stress. Burnout can occur in any profession and is not solely related to caregiving roles. Feelings of depletion, cynicism and a reduced sense of accomplishment typically characterise it. Burnout often arises from prolonged work-related stressors, such as high workloads, long hours and a lack of control or support. Compassion fatigue is more specific to the toll that caring for others can take on individuals in caregiving professions.

MORAL INJURY

Moral injury is the psychological and emotional distress resulting from actions or situations that violate an individual's deeply held moral or ethical beliefs, often causing a sense of guilt, shame or inner conflict. Unlike traditional forms of trauma that stem from external threats, moral injury arises from the internal struggle experienced when one's actions or experiences conflict with one's core values, principles, or ethical framework. This term is frequently used in contexts such as combat, health care and other high-stress environments where individuals may find themselves making decisions that contradict their sense of right and wrong.

Doctors are responsible for making important decisions about the health and wellbeing of their patients, often in the context of limited time, resources and trained staff. These decisions can be challenging, mainly when they involve life and death, requiring doctors to adhere to high professional standards. If institutional practices violate these and influence decision-making in ways that contradict a doctor's principles, it can be difficult for them to fulfil their responsibilities and maintain their integrity. This dissonance is the essence of the term moral injury.

Moral distress, a symptom of moral injury, is a feeling of unease where institutionally directed practice does not align with ethically correct action or ethical principles. The doctor may experience this in an active role of moral transgression or a passive one in witnessing others transgress. A lack of autonomy can cause moral distress for a doctor to act in the patient's best interests, insufficient resources to meet professional standards, complicity in incidents of poor care, witnessing poor standards or experience of practising against medical school and personal standards. Doctors who report moral distress or injury are more likely to work fewer hours or take early retirement, which could contribute to a vicious cycle of reduced staffing and increased risk of moral distress and injury to those left behind.[6]

Unlike formal mental health conditions such as depression or post-traumatic stress disorder (PTSD), moral injury is not classified as a mental illness. However, individuals who experience moral injuries often deal with negative thoughts about themselves or others, like feeling '*I am a terrible person*' or believing '*My bosses don't care about people's lives*'. These distressing thoughts often lead to intense emotions of shame, guilt, or disgust, which can contribute to mental health challenges, including conditions like depression, PTSD and, in severe cases, even thoughts of suicide.

Moral injury has already been documented among medical students, who have reported significant difficulties in coping with their experiences in prehospital and emergency care settings, where they were exposed to traumatic events for which they felt unprepared.

More doctors reported experiencing moral injury during the COVID-19 pandemic than before. Younger doctors, doctors from ethnic minority backgrounds and doctors with physical or mental illnesses were likelier to report such experiences.[7]

Several potential strategies can help alleviate the negative moral impacts of the current situation. Preparing all healthcare workers for the moral dilemmas they will confront during their working lives is crucial. Health care is full of ethical dilemmas, and whilst we (hope) do not experience a crisis such as a pandemic, other unexpected and difficult situations will occur, requiring clinicians to make difficult decisions quickly and sometimes without support. Adequate preparation significantly reduces the risk of mental health issues. It's essential to offer professionals a realistic assessment of their challenges, free from euphemisms and false reassurances. Failing to do so can intensify their frustration when confronted with the harsh realities.

Leaders play a vital role in helping staff navigate the morally challenging decisions that may arise in health care. One practical approach involves engaging in discussions, utilising reflective spaces such as Schwartz Rounds or Balint Groups where healthcare staff from diverse backgrounds can safely discuss the emotional and other challenges they encounter while caring for patients.

Avoidance is a common trauma symptom, so team leaders should contact staff members who claim to be 'too busy' or repeatedly 'unavailable' to participate in these discussions. Typically, individuals find support from their colleagues and immediate supervisors helpful. Those who consistently avoid such interactions or display excessive distress may benefit from a sensitive conversation and support from a qualified person, such as their team leader, a trained peer supporter or a chaplain.

COGNITIVE DISSONANCE

Linked to moral injury is the issue of cognitive dissonance. Medicine is full of committed, ethical and compassionate individuals who strive to give their patients the best possible care and maintain the highest professional standards. Yet the current socio-political environment and working conditions in which many of us work limit our ability to live up to these ideas. This creates a cognitive dissonance, which leads to disillusionment, self-doubt and depression. In psychology, cognitive dissonance is the mental discomfort (psychological stress) experienced by a person who holds two or more contradictory beliefs, ideas, or values. This discomfort is triggered by a situation in which a person's belief clashes with new evidence perceived by the person. Several psychological factors put doctors at particular risk, linked to how doctors are caught in these dilemmas.

The areas of dissonance are as follows:

- To be good doctors, doctors need to be empathic and attuned to the suffering of patients. Yet, to survive, they must develop psychological defence mechanisms to create distance between themselves and patients and become hardened to their patient's suffering.

- Doctors feel they must be 'perfect' to overcome deep-rooted self-doubt about themselves and the powers of medicine. Yet perfectionism is never achievable, and the drive to be perfect leads to doctors delivering worse care through over-treatment, constant checking and over-adherence to clinical guidelines.

- Making patients a doctor's first concern means denying their needs. Yet this risks burnout and worsening patient care. This means that doctors must put themselves first if they can put patients first.

DEPRESSION

Imagine you have fallen into a well. A deep, dark well where it is near impossible to see the light at the top of the well. You have been treading water for a while and are beginning to tire. No light indicates a climb out of the well; no clear footholds exist. Shouts for help echo off the walls. You hear cries from above very faintly, but the words are lost. You are starting to lose hope. You feel something brush against your upper body. Tiresomely, you grab the rope, and you feel tension. But you are so tired. Exhausted. You cannot keep a grip on the rope and sink back into the cold water, drenched clothes feeling heavier than before. Hope starts to wane as you wait for some sign that help is coming. You cry defiantly for help, screaming. No one is coming. Your arms and legs are in agony. The water is freezing. It is so dark.

— **Personal Account from a Foundation Year 2 Doctor**

Depression is a serious mental health condition characterised by persistent sadness, hopelessness and a lack of interest or pleasure in once-enjoyable activities. It goes beyond everyday life's normal ups and downs and impacts a person's thoughts, feelings, behaviours and overall well-being.

Common symptoms of depression include the following:

1. **Persistent sadness:** A pervasive feeling of sadness or emptiness that lasts most of the day, nearly every day.

2. **Loss of interest:** A decreased interest or pleasure in activities, hobbies and social interactions that were once enjoyable.

3. **Fatigue and lack of energy:** Feeling constantly tired and lacking the energy to perform even routine tasks.

4. **Changes in appetite or weight:** Significant changes in appetite or weight, either increased or decreased.

5. **Sleep disturbances:** Insomnia (difficulty falling or staying asleep) or hypersomnia (excessive sleepiness) are common.

6. **Feelings of worthlessness or guilt:** A persistent sense of worthlessness, guilt, or excessive self-blame.

7. **Difficulty concentrating:** Trouble focusing, making decisions, or remembering details.

8. **Physical symptoms:** Unexplained physical symptoms like headaches, abdominal pain, or other discomforts.

9. **Psychomotor agitation or retardation:** Restlessness or slowed movements and speech.

10. **Suicidal thoughts:** Persistent thoughts of death or suicide or suicidal behaviours.

Depression is a complex and multifaceted condition with various potential causes, including genetic predisposition, brain chemistry imbalances, hormonal changes, life events, trauma and environmental factors. It can affect individuals of any age, gender or background, varying from mild to severe.

Depression can significantly impact a person's daily functioning, relationships, work and overall quality of life.

Doctors, even those with training in mental health, may not always recognise the symptoms of depression in themselves. They may attribute their symptoms to the everyday stresses of working in a demanding environment and may not realise they are depressed. They might not even notice their change in mood or behaviour.

Depression clouds one's psychological vision, making focusing challenging and requiring extra energy from a depleted source to continue functioning. As the personal account describes, depression feels like darkness, a manifestation of despair.

ANXIETY

Andrew woke from a light sleep in the early hours of the morning. Drenched shirt. Racing heart. He turned off his phone's alarm, reaching over his damp sheets with a trembling hand. Andrew lived 15 minutes from the hospital but was always two hours early for the morning handover. His stomach heaved at the thought of returning to work; his heart galloped in rhythm with shallow breaths to the idea of his Rhesus shifts. 'I can't do this anymore', he said, hugging himself, crying through a mouthful of saliva, 'I need help'.

Everyone is familiar with the term 'anxiety'; no part of our daily lives can be free from it. Anxiety becomes a problem when it becomes pervasive, and the symptoms begin to interfere (for the worse) with our work, life and relationships.

An **anxiety disorder** is a mental health condition characterised by excessive and persistent feelings of worry, fear or apprehension that are disproportionate to the actual threat or situation. These feelings of anxiety can be overwhelming and interfere with a person's daily life, causing significant distress and impairing their ability to function normally.

There are several types of anxiety disorders, each with distinct features and symptoms. These include the following:

1. **Generalised anxiety disorder (GAD):** Individuals with GAD experience excessive and persistent worry about everyday concerns, such as work, health, family and finances. The worry is often challenging to control and may be accompanied by physical symptoms like restlessness, muscle tension and irritability.

2. **Panic disorder:** Panic disorder is characterised by sudden and recurrent panic attacks, which are intense episodes of fear or discomfort that reach a peak within minutes. Physical symptoms during a panic attack include heart palpitations, sweating, trembling, shortness of breath and a sense of impending doom.

3. **Specific phobias:** These involve an intense and irrational fear of a particular object, situation or activity. Common phobias include fear of heights, animals, flying and public speaking.

4. **Obsessive–compulsive disorder (OCD):** OCD is characterised by intrusive, unwanted thoughts (obsessions) that lead to repetitive behaviours or mental acts (compulsions) aimed at reducing anxiety. Despite the relief these compulsions might bring, they are often distressing and time-consuming.

5. **Post-traumatic stress disorder (PTSD):** PTSD can develop after exposure to a traumatic event, such as a severe accident, violence, or military combat. Symptoms include intrusive memories, nightmares, flashbacks and avoidance of triggers related to the trauma.

Research-wise, it is impossible to say whether anxiety is more or less as common in doctors as in the general population. Experience-wise, generalised anxiety is a common finding in the doctors seen in physician health services, either presenting alone or alongside a depressive disorder.

POST-TRAUMATIC STRESS DISORDER (PTSD)

Kamal, a 27-year-old, was attacked while on a placement in a secure psychiatric unit. The assault was severe; he genuinely believed he would be killed when his attempts to escape and get help failed. He recalls the patient's arms around his neck as he struggled to catch his breath before staff finally found him.

He received little in terms of a debrief immediately following the assault and soon rotated to a new placement. He initially struggled to sleep and was anxious around others, but he tried to 'push through' as he feared taking time off sick would extend his training. Over the next few months, he began to avoid any patient contact when he was alone with a patient. He also started to experience nightmares and hyper-arousal of his surroundings and other people. When he heard a door closing, he experienced vivid flashbacks of the assault.

PTSD is a mental health condition that can develop after a person has experienced or witnessed a traumatic or life-threatening event. While PTSD is often associated with military combat, it can occur in other contexts, including healthcare settings.

Doctors, nurses and other healthcare professionals regularly witness traumatic events, including patient deaths or dealing with significant injuries. These experiences can be upsetting, especially when involving children or other vulnerable people. Healthcare workers may also experience vicarious trauma from working with patients who have experienced trauma, which might be especially pertinent for psychiatrists and GPs who listen to the stories their patients present with, day in and day out.

Factors that may increase the risk of PTSD in doctors include high stress levels, lack of social support, feeling responsible for the outcome of patients and experiencing a lack of control over work-related events. Symptoms of PTSD can include flashbacks, nightmares, avoidance behaviours and feelings of guilt or shame.

Certain groups of doctors are associated with a higher risk of developing PTSD: Emergency physicians, doctors working in under-resourced areas, trainees, doctors involved in complaints, doctors who take personal responsibility and harbour feelings of having failed a patient. The COVID-19 pandemic revealed several additional factors raising the risk of PTSD in health workers; these stem from the ubiquitous, increased exposure to death and suffering.[8]

During the pandemic, PTSD was made worse by the conditions in which health-care workers worked. These included being separated from one's family, friends and support networks due to the risk of infection. Doctors redeployed to unfamiliar environments, sometimes poorly prepared and inadequately resourced, also added to the psychological risk of PTSD.[9]

ADDICTIONS

Eileen was one of five children raised in a strict religious family. She was all-rounded, talented at music and sports and very clever. At medical school, she excelled and was a popular and active member of the university, representing it in sports and music. She graduated top of her year. Things began to go wrong when she began her speciality training in anaesthetics. She found that the shifts affected her sleep, and she couldn't switch off when not working. She began to suffer from severe insomnia (sometimes spending the whole night up), lost weight and developed anxiety-related physical conditions – such as constant nausea, retching all night and palpitations. She also suffered from intrusive ruminations and began feeling helpless and hopeless. She did not seek help, as she did not know where to go. She felt ashamed of feeling so anxious and thought this was her fault somehow. On an occasion where she had not slept for nearly 30 hours, she took an ampoule of midazolam from work and administered it to herself via a cannula. The relief was immense when she woke hours later, re-energised. This relief was, however, short-lived, and she could only sleep when she used midazolam. Soon, she also began to inject midazolam most days, sometimes at work at the end of a list. The balloon went up when she did not turn up for work one morning, and she was found unconscious with a cannula in her arm, having taken an overdose of midazolam.

The American Association of Addiction Medicine defines **addiction** in the following manner:

> Addiction is defined as a *primary, chronic disease of brain reward, motivation, memory and related circuitry. Dysfunction in these circuits leads to characteristic biological, psychological, social and spiritual manifestations.*

This is reflected in an individual pathologically pursuing reward and relief through substance use and other behaviours. Addiction is characterised by the inability to abstain consistently, impairment in behavioural control, craving, diminished recognition of significant problems with one's behaviours and interpersonal relationships, and a dysfunctional emotional response. Like other chronic diseases, addiction often involves cycles of relapse and remission. Without treatment or engagement in recovery activities, addiction is progressive and can result in disability or premature death.

Addiction can be to substances (alcohol, drugs) or behaviours (such as gambling, sex, internet).

ICD-10

Three or more of the following presented together at some point in the last year:

1. A strong desire or sense of compulsion to take the substance.
2. Difficulties controlling substance-taking behaviour regarding its onset, termination or use levels.
3. A physiological withdrawal state when substance use has ceased or been reduced, as evidenced by the characteristic withdrawal syndrome for the substance or use of the same (or closely related) substance to relieve or avoid withdrawal symptoms.
4. Evidence of tolerance, such that increased doses of the psychoactive substance are required to achieve effects originally produced by lower doses (clear examples of this are found in alcohol- and opiate-dependent individuals who may take daily quantities sufficient to incapacitate or kill non-tolerant users).
5. Progressive neglect of alternative pleasures or interests because of psychoactive substance use; the increased time necessary to obtain or take the substance or recover from its effects.
6. Persisting with substance use despite clear evidence of overtly harmful consequences, such as harm to the liver through excessive drinking, depressive mood states consequent to periods of heavy substance use or drug-related impairment of cognitive functioning; efforts should be made to determine that the user was, or could be expected to be, aware of the nature and extent of the harm.

DSM-V

DSM-V is similar in its criteria but also determines the severity of the problem by how many symptoms are present. A minimum of two to three criteria is required to indicate a mild substance use disorder diagnosis, while four to five is moderate, and six to seven is severe.

1. Take the substance in more significant amounts or longer than you should.
2. Wanting to cut down or stop using the substance but not managing to.

3. Spending much time getting, using, or recovering from substance use.

4. Cravings and urges to use the substance.

5. Not managing to do what you should at work, home, or school because of substance use.

6. Continuing to use it, even when it causes relationship problems.

7. Giving up important social, occupational, or recreational activities because of substance use.

8. Using substances again and again, even when it puts you in danger.

9. Continuing to use, even when you know you have a physical or psychological problem that could have been caused or made worse by the substance.

10. Needing more substance to get the effect you want (tolerance).

11. The development of withdrawal symptoms can be relieved by taking more of the substance.

As an anaesthetist, Eileen, described in the vignette above, is more at risk of drug addiction than her other medical counterparts. However, studies have shown that addiction prevalence rates in doctors are similar or even much lower[10] than in the general population. Where doctors are addicted,[11,12] this is most likely to be related to alcohol.[11]

In 2017, an anaesthetist was jailed after stealing codeine from his hospital. He had done this many times before, entering the ward using his old pass to gain access. He had now been discovered with hundreds of codeine tablets in his rucksack. He had an opiate addiction. The trial judge accepted his problems were genuine but, amongst other things, said in his summing up, 'as a doctor, he should have known where to get help'. However, for many reasons, as discussed in this handbook, doctors with mental illness, and especially those with addiction, do not know where to get help. They have poor access to confidential, accessible and supportive care. They are often in denial, terrified of acknowledging that they have a problem for themselves and others. Colleagues tend not to see the obvious and often ignore the unmistakable and sometimes unpleasant stale smell of alcohol, pinpoint pupils of someone using opiates or the odd behaviour of colleagues using stimulants.

Addiction among doctors is not a new phenomenon. For example, in the late nineteenth century, most morphine users in America were doctors and estimated between 30 and 40% of medical professionals were addicted to the drug. One such eminent example is William Stewart Halsted, considered one of the greatest and most influential American surgeons. Willkie Collins, the writer of the first detective story and a doctor, struggled under the shadow of laudanum – a mixture of alcohol and opium. Sir Arthur Colon Doyle, or his fictional genius, Sherlock Holmes and many other doctors joined the growing crisis of addicted doctors. By the early twentieth century, doctors made up 90% of all people with an addiction, and 20% of the mortality amongst the profession was said to be caused by morphinism. A report published in 1924 said that of the people with a morphine addiction worldwide, 40% were doctors, and 10.0% were their wives.[13] All these data are questionable since reliable measures would have been impossible. Still, we can reasonably deduce that medical professionals were consistently the most prominent demographic group among morphine addicts in the developed Western world after the middle of the nineteenth century. This was accepted mainly until the beginning of the twentieth century as not interfering with their ability to practice. This is very different today.

Establishing accurate prevalence rates, however, is challenging because assured anonymity may not sufficiently guarantee participants' safety, potentially jeopardising their employment status. UK studies are now over 30 years old and are either based on self-reported data, which could lead to underestimations of actual occurrences or inferred from treatment samples. These studies also occurred before the significant changes implemented after the Dame Janet Smith Inquiry in 2000 (held after the murderous actions of the GP Harold Shipman, who had been a pethidine addict early in his career) brought about substantial shifts in how doctors handle controlled substances. Data from the General Medical Council (GMC) between 2005 and 2019 show that just over 2,000 doctors in the UK had criminal records (against more than 200,000 on the register). More than 50% of crimes were for vehicle-related offences such as dangerous driving (speeding, drunk or drug driving) and motoring offences (driving without insurance or tax). Whilst it is only speculation, many of these are likely related to alcohol and drug use – this means treatable mental health problems if the individual had sought help before the criminal incident.

Barriers to seeking help for doctors who have an addiction disorder

Even given the problems faced by doctors with mental illness in seeking help, they are compounded when their problem is related to addiction.

Addicted doctors endure almost universal negative attitudes from colleagues, the public and those who have jurisdiction over them. This leads to secrecy for fear of exposure, and denial is common. For example, a doctor who reports, 'I don't drink much more than anyone else', can hold onto this belief despite being caught on a drink-drive charge. Or the junior doctor 'dabbling' in drugs, 'All my friends do it; it's just to let off some steam, only at the weekends', but must miss work on a Monday due to the 'come down'. Or the anaesthetist 'It was only once; I was stressed, the Fentanyl calmed me down. It won't happen again' but finds they can't resist the open medicines cabinet at work. Fear and isolation lead to doctors often presenting in a crisis, following a drink-drive offence, or sadly, the first indication that the doctor is addicted is a failed or successful suicide attempt.

Problems linked to addiction

The use of drugs, alcohol and addiction brings a host of problems. Addicted doctors are more likely to be involved in criminal behaviour. Either through theft of medicines or goods to pay for them, drunk or drug driving, aggressive or violent behaviour whilst intoxicated, or obtaining medicines through fraudulent prescriptions. Not surprisingly, they are more likely to be involved in disciplinary and regulatory processes. Doctors found using illegal drugs are often subjected to multiple jeopardy – with sanctions taken against them by their employer, regulator and usually the police. The various legal, regulatory and disciplinary processes can take years, affecting the doctor's personal, professional and financial lives.

Why do doctors develop an addiction disorder?

The aetiology of addictions in doctors is multi-factorial, including genetic predisposition, personality factors (for example, risk takers), stress at work, co-morbid mental illness, family stress, grief, an injury or accident at work, pain and a non-specific drift into heavy drinking. These are like the factors found in the general population. What is different for doctors is their work environment (high stress, low tolerance for failure, culture of 'name and blame') and easy access to prescribed and non-prescribed medication.

Where addiction is found among doctors, certain specialities have consistently been more vulnerable, with an over-representation of emergency doctors and psychiatrists using multiple substances.[14] Studies of American physicians found that family doctors (GPs), internal medicine doctors, anaesthetists, emergency medicine doctors and psychiatrists accounted for over 50% of the cohort, with anaesthetists alone accounting for almost 11% of addicted doctors.[13] Most studies looking at addicted doctors show a pattern of predominately alcohol use, followed by misuse of opiates and stimulants.[15]

A higher proportion of anaesthetists compared to other doctors report intravenous drug use. Additional risk factors for anaesthetists include[16] the following:

- Direct contact with drugs.
- Daily exposure to highly potent and addictive opioids and sedatives.
- Drugs are immediately available.

- Only a small volume is required, so it is easy to divert from the anaesthetic room.

- Students with an addiction problem may favour anaesthesia as a speciality due to its easy drug access.

When opiates are the problem, they are more likely to be self-prescribed or stolen from hospital stock rather than obtained from 'the street' or *the dark web*.

A recent trend, especially amongst the male gay community, is the use of club drugs.[17] Club drugs are a group of psychoactive drugs often used by young people at clubs, concerts and parties. These drugs are known for altering mood and perception and can produce various effects, including euphoria, increased energy and altered consciousness. Some common club drugs include MDMA (known as 'Ecstasy'), GHB, ketamine and LSD. These drugs can have severe effects on physical and mental health. Doctors might be even more reluctant when drugs enhance sexual activity.

Treatment of addiction disorder

Several attempts have been made to encourage addicted doctors into treatment. In the UK, as early as the 1970s, the psychiatrist Max Glatt, a survivor of the Holocaust, set up a group for doctors where they could meet, share their experiences, and garner support from each other. This was the precursor of what we now know as the British Doctors & Dentists Group (BDDG). He noted how well doctors did once in treatment, with many becoming abstinent and being able to return to work.

In North America, as a response to their growing numbers of addicted doctors and for a genuine desire to bridge the gap between sanction and care, the American Medical Association encouraged the expansion of Medical Professionals' Health Programs (now called Physician Health Programs) to '*improve physician wellness and eliminate any barriers that stand in the way of physicians accessing needed mental health-care services*'.

Practitioner Health (PH) was established in 2008 to provide confidential help to doctors and dentists with mental health and addiction issues. The service was set up following two unique events. The first, as mentioned, was the death through suicide of a young psychiatrist who had severe post-natal psychosis. Before she killed herself, she also killed her three-month-old baby.

The second and very different event was the murderous activities of the GP, Harold Shipman, who early in his career had been addicted to pethidine and was thought to have then become addicted to killing. The inquiry following his murders led to a tightening of doctor's access to controlled drugs but also recognised the need for them, if addicted, to have access to confidential care.

In different ways, both events led to funding being found to establish PH.

Changes in presentations to Practitioner Health (2008–2022)

At the start of the service in 2008, around one-third of all presentations were doctors with addiction, mainly older male doctors with alcohol addiction. However, as the years progressed, there has been a year-on-year drop in the proportion of patients attending with any form of drug or alcohol addiction, and as of 2022, at around 7% of all presentations. Whilst alcohol still predominates, increasing numbers over the years have presented with opiates, methamphetamines and other psychostimulants.

The drop in overall numbers might be related to doctors having fewer opportunities for unrestricted access to drugs of abuse since stricter prescribing rules following the inquiry led by Dame Janet Smith into the actions of the GP, Harold Shipman and the use and abuse of controlled drugs. Nowadays, even the ability to self-prescribe drugs such as benzodiazepines raises concerns, let alone if the doctor is trying to obtain drugs such as codeine, morphine, or other strong opiates. This means that the opportunity for doctors to become addicted through better access to drugs has been significantly curtailed, except in specific fields such as anaesthetics, surgery and emergency medicine (where there is access to onsite drugs at work, albeit strict monitoring protocols) and general practice. It might also be due to doctors presenting before use becomes problematic and entrenched.

The earlier high prevalence is likely an unmet need, especially as the first cohorts of doctors tended to be male, over 50 years old, with long-standing alcohol dependence.

The treatment of addiction will be discussed more fully later in this handbook.

PERSONALITY DISORDER

A **personality disorder** is a mental health condition characterised by enduring patterns of thoughts, emotions, behaviours and interpersonal functioning that deviate significantly from cultural norms and societal expectations. These patterns often lead to distress, impairment in daily life and difficulties in forming and maintaining relationships. Personality disorders typically emerge in adolescence or early adulthood and remain relatively stable.

Personality and personality disorders are not the same. Everyone has different personality traits – some of which become exaggerated at different times. A personality is an individual's characteristic way of behaving, experiencing life and perceiving and interpreting themselves, others, events and situations.

Personality disorders can be accompanied by disruptive behaviour at work or professional misconduct, such as boundary violations. Such performance transgressions are often taken as a proxy for a personality disorder. A study from the University of Florida has classified disruptive behaviours of doctors into three levels:

- Mild offences, such as poor documentation and frequent lateness.

- Persistent low-level offences or a single incident, such as an aggressive act or sexually inappropriate conduct.

- Behaviours carrying a significant risk of harm to staff and patients, such as ignoring warnings of medical errors potentially leading to severe incidents.[18]

Disruptive behaviours are considered present in 3%–5% of doctors. However, their impact may be significant, with over 90% of doctors and nurses experiencing such behaviours in the workplace.[19] These doctors often avoid investigation or sanctions. Staff are often reluctant to report their behaviour, and even when they do, their concerns are rarely acted on. Staff also might wrongly try to protect a colleague, fearing that if they do raise any alarm, the colleague might suffer in their career development. There is often a conspiracy of silence. At the organisational level, senior staff often look the other way if they are made aware of a senior member of their clinical staff exhibiting poor behaviour. They might also need better policies and practices to deal with poor behaviour. The disruptive clinician might escape investigation due to their working practices – working as a locum or moving rotations frequently. Large impersonal teams also act as a barrier to addressing disruptive behaviour.

Disruptive behaviours amongst healthcare professionals significantly threaten patient safety and quality of care.[20]

AUTISM

Autism is not a mental illness, though autistic people are more likely to develop mental health problems. It is a complex, lifelong neurodevelopmental condition that changes how an individual experiences the world and communicates with others.

Individuals on the autism spectrum exhibit distinct strengths and challenges, including hyperfocus, differences in sensory perception, special interests and anxiety. It is characterised by enduring communication, interaction, socialisation and behaviour variations.

The global and UK prevalence of autism is estimated at least 1%, with research in Northern Ireland indicating a prevalence of around 5% among school-aged children. The rise in diagnosis rates in recent years can be attributed to increased awareness about autism, improved screening methods and enhanced diagnostic accuracy.[21]

Traditionally, autism research focused on deficits and challenges. However, a shift towards the neurodiversity paradigm has gained momentum. This perspective challenges the pathologising approach by recognising that autism is not an inherent flaw but a set of differences. Aligned with the social model of disability, this paradigm considers social, cultural, political and environmental factors as contributors to contextual disability.

Specific attributes commonly associated with autism, such as attention to detail and pattern recognition, can be advantageous in medical professionals. As autism awareness and diagnosis increase, more medical students and practitioners may discover their autism spectrum condition. These realisations can occur at any point during training or careers, sometimes in response to challenges in demanding clinical environments.

Some colleagues may be sceptical that a qualified physician could be autistic, reinforcing negative stereotypes. Negotiating such an environment could lead to internalised ableism and hinder disclosure. A study published in 2023 revealed that only 63% of employed autistic adults openly acknowledged their autism. This issue is significant in the medical field, where disclosing any disability is often avoided due to fear of appearing weak.[22]

Recognising intersectionality and diversification within the medical workforce has gained momentum. The UK has generated supportive guidelines on diversity and inclusion. These guidelines underscore the rights of autistic individuals regarding reasonable accommodations in education and employment, as mandated by law. However, achieving a genuinely inclusive workforce remains an ongoing endeavour.

Helpful information about the impact of neurodiversity is provided by the General Medical Council and Medical Schools Council, as with the links below.

- General Medical Council (2019). Welcomed and valued: Supporting disabled learners in medical education and training [online]. Available at: *https:// www.gmc-uk. org/-/media/latest-welcomed-and-valued-full-guidance.pdf*
- Medical Schools Council (2021). Active inclusion: Challenging exclusions in medical education [online]. Available at: *https://www.medschools.ac.uk/ media/2918/active- inclusion-challenging-exclusions-in-medical-education.pdf*

While there is limited research on autism in the medical profession, there is growing recognition of the need to support doctors with this condition and ensure they can thrive in their careers.

As awareness and diagnosis of autism are growing, more medical students and doctors may be discovering they are autistic, and this may occur at any stage through their training or working lives.[23]

A study involving those with a formal diagnosis or self-diagnosis of autism found that half had engaged in self-harming behaviour, and over three-quarters had considered suicide, compared with lifetime suicidal ideation rates of under 10% in the general population.[24]

Doctors with autism may face challenges in their professional lives. For example, they may struggle with communication and social interactions with colleagues and patients, affecting their ability to work in a team or build rapport with patients. They may also experience sensory sensitivities, which can be particularly challenging in a hospital or clinic's fast-paced and often chaotic environment. Shirley Moore, a doctor who was dismissed from the NHS following a long absence of depression and anxiety, was eventually diagnosed with autism, thus giving her an insight into why she experienced difficulties as a trainee.[25]

Moore writes,

> *I always felt I was working far harder than my peers to keep afloat. I needed details and explanations that were unnecessary to others, and it took me longer to become confident in procedures and my abilities. I felt stupid. Appearing normal was exhausting, but I felt like an outsider and did not fit in with my peers and colleagues.*

Doctors with autism can also bring additional strengths and perspectives to their work. For example, they may be detail-oriented, have excellent memory recall and can focus for extended periods. They may also have a unique understanding of the experiences of patients with autism and be able to provide more empathetic and tailored care.

There are possible links between autism and speciality choice. A speciality such as anaesthesia, which is procedure-based, solution-focused and advocates strict adherence to protocols and routines, may benefit from doctors with autistic traits.

Diagnosis can be challenging as autism is rarely considered in the differential diagnosis when a doctor presents with a mental illness, and a lifetime of masking to fit in can often obscure the signs. Missed diagnoses or making the wrong diagnosis are common, particularly in women. Anxiety, depression, or substance misuse are often the presenting conditions. Patients with autism are often misdiagnosed as having bipolar disorder, obsessive–compulsive disorder, schizophrenia, or personality disorders.

ATTENTION DEFICIT HYPERACTIVITY DISORDER (ADHD)

As a child, I was incredibly hyperactive, and I still am. I vividly recall a hilarious family anecdote where I had consumed much coke (soda) at a party. Upon returning home, I turned into a Tasmanian Devil-type figure. I tore up my mother's shirts and knocked myself unconscious, jumping off my bunk bed. Despite my hyperactivity, I was a bright child who loved to read, and my dad encouraged me to channel my energy by playing rugby.

My mother took me to see a kindly old GP who ultimately inspired me to become a doctor. He advised my mother to watch my diet closely and avoid caffeine, chocolate, e-numbers and food colourings; I am now a psychiatrist and have found techniques to help me manage my hyperactivity. During memory clinic assessments that could take up to an hour and a half, I jiggled my leg under the table, which annoyed an elderly patient. So, I developed a new technique of drumming my fingers under my leg while using my other hand for the assessment. It's a strategy that works for me.

If I want to watch a film longer than an hour, I need to take a break and pace around before continuing. My family understands my need to move around, and my former girlfriend was my diary, caretaker and organiser. She helped me shield the worst effects of my attention deficit hyperactivity disorder (ADHD). I miss her deeply sometimes.

— Patient at PH

ADHD is a neurodevelopmental disorder that affects attention, impulsivity and hyperactivity. ADHD is becoming increasingly common among all ages, genders and professional groups. It affects around 2% of UK adults. It is commonly recognised as a specific learning difference due to the impact of inattentive and hyperactive symptoms on performance at school, university and work. It is often not diagnosed until adulthood – sufferers are often first misdiagnosed with depression and anxiety disorders during their teenage years, induced by the struggle of compensating for an unrecognised neurodevelopmental disorder.

While there is limited research on ADHD in doctors, studies suggest that doctors with ADHD may face challenges in their professional lives. For example, they might struggle to manage their symptoms in a high-stress and fast-paced work environment. Symptoms of ADHD, such as difficulty focusing, impulsivity and disorganisation, can make it challenging to keep up with the demands of a busy medical practice. This can lead to feelings of being overwhelmed, burnout and frustration. They might find certain aspects of their job, such as administrative tasks or maintaining patient records, which require a high level of organisation and attention to detail, very difficult. Accounts from doctors have been written regarding their experiences as students and doctors with ADHD. The themes covered include the stigma associated with the diagnosis, episodes of anxiety and depression and an improvement following the correct diagnosis and treatment plan.

Doctors with ADHD can also bring strengths to their work. For example, they may be exceptionally skilled at multi-tasking and able to quickly shift their attention between different tasks or patients. They may also be more creative and able to think outside of the box regarding problem-solving.

There are increasing concerns that ADHD might be overdiagnosed. Whilst there are no studies on overdiagnosis among doctors, there is evidence that overdiagnosis and over-treatment are prevalent in children and adolescents. Overdiagnosis and over-treatment in themselves might have negative consequences for the individual.[26]

Evidential gaps remain, and future research is needed on the long-term benefits and harms of diagnosing and treating ADHD in people, in particular, those with milder symptoms; therefore, practitioners should be mindful of these knowledge gaps, especially when identifying these individuals and to ensure safe and equitable practice and policy.

A quality improvement exercise at PH has been carried out at the time of writing, though it still needs to be completed. Early findings, however, indicate that 30%–40% of all new presentations to the service (around 2,000 individuals in total during the study period) scored positively when completing an internationally recognised tool for ADHD (Adult ASRS). More work is being done to indicate whether this finding is an artefact of the underlying mental illness (anxiety, depression) or indicates exceptionally high levels of ADHD in this treatment group.

BIPOLAR AFFECTIVE DISORDER (BPAD)

Bipolar disorder, previously known as *manic–depressive disorder*, is a mental health condition characterised by extreme mood, energy and activity shifts. These mood shifts, known as episodes, range from depressive lows to manic or hypomanic highs. Bipolar disorder can significantly impact a person's daily life, relationships and overall well-being.

There are several types of bipolar disorder, each with varying degrees of severity and symptom patterns:

- **Bipolar I disorder:** In this type, individuals experience at least one manic episode that lasts at least one week and often requires hospitalisation. Depressive episodes may also occur.

- **Bipolar II disorder:** People with bipolar II experience one or more major depressive episodes and at least one hypomanic episode (a milder form of mania) lasting at least four consecutive days.

- **Cyclothymic disorder:** This involves periods of hypomanic symptoms and depressive symptoms that last for at least two years (one year in children and adolescents). The symptoms are less severe than in full-blown episodes of mania or depression.

- **Other specified and unspecified bipolar and related disorders:** These categories include symptoms that do not fit the criteria of the above types but still involve significant mood disturbances.

Symptoms of bipolar disorder vary depending on the mood episode:

- **Manic episode:** During manic episodes, individuals experience heightened energy, euphoria, grandiosity, decreased need for sleep, rapid speech, racing thoughts, impulsivity and risky behaviours such as excessive spending or engaging in reckless activities.

- **Hypomanic episode:** Hypomania is a less severe form of mania characterised by increased energy, elevated mood and heightened creativity. Individuals may be productive and engaging, but these episodes are less extreme than full manic episodes.

- **Depressive episode:** Depressive episodes involve persistent sadness, hopelessness, loss of interest in activities, changes in appetite and sleep patterns, fatigue, difficulty concentrating and thoughts of death or suicide.

Bipolar disorder can be challenging to live with as it impacts a person's daily functioning but does not preclude someone from having a medical career. Symptoms of bipolar disorder can include periods of elevated mood (mania or hypomania) and periods of depressed mood. The severity of these symptoms can vary from person to person and change over time.

There are no definitive studies regarding the prevalence of bipolar disorders among doctors; however, like many chronic severe health conditions, it is reasonable to consider a prevalence somewhat lower than the general population based on the assumption that medical training tends to select people with more severe forms of disability. Bipolar affective disorder accounts for less than 3% of all the patients registered at PH.

PH probably has the largest cohort of doctors with BPAD in a single service. A full audit of patients was conducted in 2018 when 70 patients with this diagnosis received treatment from the service.[27] Overall, GPs made up 52% and psychiatrists 15% of the patient cohort, with an average age of 45. Men and women were evenly distributed. Patients at the service either have this diagnosis at presentation or the diagnosis was made following a clinical assessment (sometimes over many sessions). The criteria used for diagnosis are those laid down by best practice (ICD-10).

The Bipolar Doc, an NHS doctor who left the profession and retrained as a primary school teacher, has written her account of suffering from the disorder, her struggles coping with a busy paediatric job and her decision to leave and become a teacher.[28] Her poignant and honest writings follow her journey and the impact of her illness on her life, her identity and her ability to work as a doctor. She talks about the stigma and shame associated with admitting vulnerability but the relief when she was able to be open and honest with colleagues and friends. Her writings are some of the most powerful descriptions of what it means to be unwell, to lose an identity, but to come through this and find solace in another profession. She gives her experience of 'opening up' to patients.

> *All too often in the healthcare sector, we refer to vulnerability as a negative attribute. We are expected to pick ourselves up, brush ourselves off and get on with things. Stigma silences us.*

> *Clearly there is a boundary when it comes to sharing our own struggles with patients. After all, we remain the professional in the relationship and, as such, need to be aware of how the disclosure may impact on that. Revealing insecurity doesn't have to be done by spelling things out though. Thoughtful questioning and understanding can be sufficient to help the patient feel valued.*

> *However, opening can leave us feeling exposed. I was convinced that I would get into trouble for my behaviour. I worried about it for days. What if someone at work found out? What if they thought I could no longer be a good doctor?*

> *It turns out nothing happened. Of course, it didn't. I did nothing wrong. Being true to ourselves isn't always such a bad thing.*

Bipolar disorders have a chronic course and are associated with markedly elevated premature mortality. One of the contributors to the decreased life expectancy is suicide, and its rate is approximately 10–30 times higher than in the general population, with up to 20% of (mostly untreated) people with BPAD ending their life by suicide and 20–60% having attempted at least one in their lifetime.[29]

SUICIDE

Suicide is not a mental illness, though it is often the result of one. As with the general population, the reasons why someone takes their own life are often related to un (or under) treated depression, bipolar disorder, or substance misuse. Suicide is also a risk for any professional group with ready access to the means, including doctors and their access to drugs (and the skills to use them). The most frequent method of suicide in doctors is self-poisoning (51%), with ready access to prescription medications a risk factor for individual doctors.[30] Anaesthetists, community health doctors, GPs and psychiatrists have higher suicide rates than general hospital doctors.[31,32] Female doctors have higher rates of suicide compared with the general population and other professional groups. Data from Australia show that risk is higher in female doctors (146% elevated risk compared to the general population for female doctors *versus* 26% for male doctors).[33]

Suicide will be discussed in greater depth later in this handbook.

4

Why doctors become mentally unwell

Mental illness in doctors is not a new phenomenon, but the current levels of unhappiness and disillusionment are concerning. It can be challenging for those outside the medical profession to understand why doctors are experiencing such high rates of mental illness, considering the host of protective factors they share. They are intelligent, tend not to have been brought up in the care system or have had unstable accommodation (such as living in bed-and-breakfasts), and even the most isolated doctor works within a team structure. Doctors have high-status jobs, a good and reasonably stable income and, even if it sometimes doesn't seem so, are well respected. This does not mean that doctors do not have their fill of life events – and it might have been early adverse trauma (such as exposure to illness, death, or disability) which drew them into the caring profession in the first place.

The reasons why doctors experience high rates of unhappiness and distress are multifaceted and complex. Some factors are related to the nature of the job itself, such as the emotional toll of working closely with suffering patients. Other factors stem from the characteristics of those who become doctors, including the tendency towards perfectionism and high levels of self-criticism.

Let us look at some of these in detail in the following sections.

PERSONALITY

Personality refers to a unique and enduring pattern of thoughts, emotions, behaviours and characteristics that distinguish an individual from others. It is how a person thinks, feels and acts across various situations and contexts. Personality is relatively stable but can evolve and change as a person experiences life events and personal growth.

Many theories attempt to explain the underlying mechanisms that shape and influence personality. These range from psychodynamic interpretations, such as Sigmund Freud's psychoanalytic theory, to contemporary approaches, such as humanistic, cognitive and social-cognitive theories. Each theory offers insights into how personality develops, the role of genetics and environment and how people perceive and interact with the world.

Doctors may be at additional risk because they are *chosen* for those personality factors that foster the antecedents of burnout, which also attract the individual to a medical career. These include altruism, perfectionism and obsessiveness.

Altruism refers to the selfless concern for the well-being and welfare of others. It involves acting to benefit others without expecting personal gain or reward. Altruistic actions can encompass various behaviours, from helping those in need and making sacrifices to assisting others and demonstrating compassion and empathy. Altruism often involves placing the needs and interests of others above one's own, and it can be motivated by a genuine desire to alleviate suffering, promote fairness or contribute positively to the lives of others and society.

Perfectionism is a personality trait or characteristic marked by an individual's constant striving for flawlessness and setting exceedingly high standards for themselves and their work. Perfectionists tend to have a strong desire to achieve and maintain an exceptionally high level of performance, often holding themselves to unrealistic expectations. They might believe that any outcome short of perfection is unacceptable and can be overly critical of themselves when they perceive that they have fallen short.

Perfectionism can manifest in various areas of life, such as academia, work, personal relationships and even hobbies. While striving for excellence can have positive outcomes, excessive or unhealthy perfectionism can lead to negative consequences. These might include heightened stress and anxiety due to the pressure to meet unrealistic goals, a fear of failure, difficulty completing tasks due to overly critical self-evaluation and even dissatisfaction despite accomplishing impressive achievements.

There are different forms of perfectionism, including:

1. **Self-oriented perfectionism:** This involves setting high personal standards and being critical of oneself when those standards are not met. These individuals often experience significant internal pressure to excel.

2. **Other-oriented perfectionism:** This form revolves around setting high standards for others and expecting them to meet them. Individuals with other-oriented perfectionism may feel frustrated or disappointed when others do not meet their expectations.

3. **Socially prescribed perfectionism:** This type is characterised by the feeling that others have high expectations for themselves. These individuals may believe they must meet these to gain approval and avoid criticism.

As said, perfectionism can have positive and negative effects, and finding a healthy balance is crucial. Perfectionism can involve setting reasonable goals, striving for excellence while accepting that mistakes and imperfections are a natural part of life and coping with setbacks constructively. On the other hand, it can lead to burnout, anxiety disorders, depression and a diminished overall quality of life.

Perfectionism can lead to a vicious cycle where individuals feel pressured to work harder and longer to achieve their high standards, ultimately leading to physical and mental exhaustion. This can have severe consequences beyond the workplace, including strain on personal relationships, physical health problems and reduced overall well-being. The relentless pursuit of perfection can lead to burnout, anxiety and depression, as well as impaired clinical judgement and decision-making. Perfectionism can also lead to a reluctance to seek help or admit mistakes, ultimately harming patient care.

A **compulsive triad** of doubt, guilt and an exaggerated sense of responsibility, common among doctors, adds to their vulnerability.[34]

Doctors also score higher than population averages on personality measures such as **conscientiousness, extraversion and agreeableness**.[35]

PSYCHOLOGICAL 'EGO-DEFENCES'

Becoming a doctor involves more than just absorbing the information needed to diagnose and treat disease. Doctors must learn the profession's rules, customs and practices, which have evolved over millennia. From the first day at medical school, students need to understand these rules and, in so doing, become part of their chosen group or tribe, medicine. This learning happens not just in the formal lectures, ward rounds or tutorials but as part of the informal, hidden, uncodified curriculum in the spaces in between. Individuals are taught to conform to ways of behaving, speaking and dressing; importantly, they also learn and adopt the rules of self-sacrifice. Individuals are largely unaware of this process and how they take on the persona of 'the doctor' from distressing experiences. They are also taught how to protect themselves from difficult emotional experiences. Physically, through wearing protective personal equipment such as masks, gloves and gowns, the same is true psychologically as we develop psychological protection against work trauma.

Sarah is a respected surgeon with a reputation for her exceptional skills and expertise. However, beneath her professional façade, she harbours a deep-seated fear of failure and a need for control. One day, she is due to perform complex surgery on a critically ill patient. As the surgery approaches, she starts experiencing mounting anxiety and doubts about her abilities. She begins questioning whether she can successfully carry out such a demanding procedure. She pushes these thoughts from her mind, tells herself she is 'the best' and 'has never failed' and strides confidently into the operating theatre, ready to take control.

Unbeknownst to her conscious mind, Sarah activates the defence mechanism of 'omnipotence' to cope with her insecurities. This is a psychological defence mechanism characterised by an unconscious belief or desire to be all-powerful, infallible, and capable of overcoming any challenge. A '**psychological ego-defence**', also known as a *defence mechanism*, is a psychological concept that refers to individuals' unconscious mental processes to protect themselves from distressing thoughts, feelings, or situations. These defence mechanisms operate at an unconscious level and help individuals manage internal conflicts and maintain emotional equilibrium, even if they might distort reality or hinder personal growth.

These defence mechanisms were first introduced by Sigmund Freud, the founder of psychoanalysis, and later expanded upon by other psychologists.

In the operating room, her defence mechanism manifests as an exaggerated display of confidence and control. She takes charge, dismissing any input or concerns from her surgical team, convinced that only she knows what is best for the patient. She refuses to acknowledge the possibility of complications or unforeseen challenges, as doing so would shatter her illusion of invincibility.

Some common psychological defences that doctors might use include[36] the following:

- **Intellectualisation:** Distancing oneself from emotions by focusing on the facts and logic of a situation. This is common among doctors and manifests when doctors present a case's 'hard facts', ignoring any underlying emotional issues that might affect them in the patient's care. For example, a neonatal death review following the death of an infant might skip over the involvement with parents, the impact of the death on the staff, and any feelings associated with the baby's death.

- **Compartmentalisation:** Separating different aspects of one's life, such as work and personal life, to avoid emotional conflicts.

- **Altruism:** Focusing on helping others to avoid negative emotions. Altruism can become martyrdom, with doctors neglecting their own needs or those of their families.

- **Denial:** This is a core feature of many doctors who attend treatment services and is particularly prevalent in addiction. These doctors (as with their non-medical counterparts) often deny that they use substances or are intoxicated until there is incontrovertible evidence.

- **Humour:** Using humour to diffuse stressful situations and reduce anxiety. Humour is often employed in some of medicine's most stressful, traumatic areas, which is no coincidence. It allows health professionals to discharge some of the emotional energy without connecting too deeply to the pain provoked.

- **Suppression:** Deliberately pushing negative thoughts, feelings and memories out of one's awareness.

- **Omnipotence:** The individual responds to emotional conflict or internal and external stressors by acting superior to others as if one possesses extraordinary powers, abilities, control or influence over a situation or environment. This defence mechanism is to cope with overwhelming fear and anxiety by convincing themselves they have complete control over their surroundings and events. Omnipotence can lead to individuals projecting their vulnerabilities onto patients, taking on the 'galloping helper' role as a defence against their own needs. Unchecked can also lead to a distorted sense of reality and interpersonal difficulties if the person's behaviour becomes controlling or domineering.

These defence mechanisms can be adaptive by temporarily relieving emotional distress. Psychological defences, like other forms of protection, when employed immaturely, prematurely, or excessively, can quickly become an impediment and even pathological. Whilst they can be helpful in the short term, relying on them too much can lead to emotional distancing and decreased resilience. For example, denial can lead to rejection of vulnerability, with a loss of insight and perspective. It can even lead to denial of responsibility for an error or significant event at work, as doctors may instead blame others or outside forces, including the regulator or inspectorate.

Returning to Sarah, and her operation is going differently than planned.

During the surgery, Sarah encounters unexpected difficulties and becomes increasingly rigid in her approach. She makes her team follow her instructions without question, dismissing their suggestions or concerns as irrelevant. Despite indications that her initial strategy may not work optimally, she adamantly persists, unwilling to admit the possibility of being wrong.

As the procedure progresses, the mounting tension in the room becomes palpable. Her insistence on maintaining an image of infallibility hinders effective teamwork and collaboration. Her colleagues feel excluded, leading to a breakdown in communication and potential errors that could have been avoided with a more open and collaborative approach.

While the defence mechanism of omnipotence momentarily shields her from her deep-seated insecurities, it ultimately creates a barrier to growth, learning and effective problem-solving. She jeopardises the surgery's success and her patient's well-being by denying the potential for vulnerability and her team's valuable contributions.

COGNITIVE DISTORTIONS

Cognitive theory gained ground in the later part of the twentieth century, led by the work of the psychiatrist and founder of cognitive behaviour therapy, Aaron Beck. He redefined the psychoanalytic model of ego-defences in his theory of cognitive distortions. Cognitive distortions can make the seemingly intolerable

tolerable and vice versa. Cognitive distortions, also known as *thinking errors* or *irrational thoughts*, are biased or distorted thinking patterns that can negatively impact our perception of ourselves, others and the world around us. These distortions often contribute to negative emotions and can interfere with our well-being. Cognitive distortions are commonly associated with various mental health conditions, including anxiety and depression.

Common cognitive distortions are as follows:

1. **All-or-nothing thinking ('Black-and-White Thinking'):** This distortion involves seeing things in extreme terms without considering any middle ground. It is either 'all good' or 'all bad', with no room for shades of grey. For example, if a doctor makes a minor mistake during a procedure, they might believe they are a complete failure in everything they do. One is either an exceptional doctor who can fix any problem or a complete failure incapable of making a difference. This rigid thinking pattern leaves no space for acknowledging the complex nature of medical practice and the factors beyond one's control.

2. **Overgeneralisation:** This distortion involves drawing broad conclusions based on limited or isolated incidents. It occurs when we take one negative experience and assume it represents a never-ending pattern. For instance, a doctor may make an error in diagnosis and then believe they are always wrong in their medical assessments.

3. **Mental filtering:** This distortion refers to selectively focusing only on the negative aspects of a situation while ignoring any positive aspects, dwelling solely on the negative. For example, a doctor may receive numerous positive patient feedbacks but focus only on one negative comment, feeling as though they are incompetent.

4. **Mind reading:** This distortion involves assuming we know what others think without concrete evidence and attributing negative thoughts or intentions to others without considering alternative explanations. For instance, a doctor might believe their colleagues are judging them for taking time off for mental health reasons, even though there is no direct evidence for this assumption.

5. **Catastrophising:** This distortion involves magnifying or exaggerating the potential adverse outcomes of a situation and imagining the worst-case scenario. It often involves irrational fears and imagining catastrophic consequences that are unlikely to occur. For example, a doctor might exaggerate a small mistake and believe it will significantly harm the patient and ruin their career.

6. **Emotional reasoning:** This distortion occurs when one assumes their emotions reflect reality or accurately represent the truth. They believe it must be true if they feel confident, disregarding contradictory evidence. For instance, a doctor may feel anxious about difficult surgery and conclude that they cannot perform it successfully.

7. **Personalisation:** This distortion assumes we are solely responsible for events or situations beyond our control. We tend to blame ourselves for adverse outcomes, even when other factors are involved. For example, doctors may blame themselves for a patient's poor health outcome, even due to factors outside their control.

ORGANISATIONAL DEFENCES

It is not just individuals who develop psychological defences to cope with the emotional task of delivering care. Organisations also establish structures and practices that protect those within them from anxiety. As with individual ones, organisational reasons give the illusion of certainty and safety and protect from being overwhelmed by emotions. The seminal work of Isobel Menzies-Lyth helped to describe what she called social (institutional) defences, social as they are created by the organisation in which they work. She was a British academic who, from a background in economics and experimental psychology, joined the Tavistock Institute in London, where she qualified as a psychoanalyst in 1954.[37] She drew attention to the stress nurses experienced who were engaged in incredibly distasteful tasks; those connected to death and sexuality were found to be most disturbing. The defence mechanisms she described are like those seen in individuals who experienced: depersonalisation, denial and detachment. She argued that practices such as handovers, frequent ward rounds, use of rigid protocols, systems of allocating tasks and responsibilities and the rule of referring to a patient in abstract ways, such as *'the liver in Bed 10'*, were aimed at discouraging attachment and engagement with the patient. Once split off from ordinary consciousness, the left-over anxiety is acted out through either idealising or denigrating those who have taken the unpalatable tasks away.

Common organisational defences seen in hospitals and other health organisations include the following:

- **Rituals and routines:** Using practices, routines and standard operating procedures (SOPs) that provide stability and predictability, these repetitive patterns help manage anxiety and maintain control within the organisation.

- **Role segregation:** Organisational roles and responsibilities are often clearly defined and separated, which can create boundaries and prevent emotional overload. By compartmentalising tasks and functions, individuals can focus on specific work areas without becoming overwhelmed by the broader organisational context.

- **Task focus:** Organisations often emphasise task-oriented activities and objectives, which can distract from emotional or interpersonal issues. A strong emphasis on tasks and productivity can minimise opportunities for emotional expression and interpersonal conflict.

- **Depersonalisation:** Organisations may adopt practices and structures that depersonalise interactions and relationships. This minimises emotional involvement and maintains a professional distance, helping individuals manage anxieties and potential conflicts arising from emotional connections.

- **Idealisation and denial:** Organisational cultures may idealise specific values, such as teamwork, efficiency, or productivity, while denying or ignoring underlying emotional or relational issues. Idealisation is a defence against acknowledging and addressing potential weaknesses or conflicts within the organisation.

- **Splitting:** Organisations may break, separating issues into extremes or dichotomies. This defence mechanism simplifies complex situations, avoiding the discomfort of dealing with ambiguity or conflicting viewpoints.

- **Resistance to change:** Particularly if change threatens established routines or challenges existing power dynamics.

Understanding and recognising these organisational defence mechanisms can illuminate an organisation's hidden dynamics and emotional challenges.

CHOOSING MEDICINE WRONGLY

An individual's choice to be a doctor can influence their susceptibility to developing a mental illness. Understanding these can provide insight into the individual's challenges and potential sources of stress or burnout.

For example, this is Alex story:

Alex grew up in a household with a family member who battled a chronic illness; his mother had severe rheumatoid arthritis. Witnessing her suffering, its impact on their family and the caring doctors provided, he decided to become a doctor. During medical school, he excelled academically. However, as he progressed through his clinical rotations, it became apparent that his motivation for becoming a doctor, rooted in unresolved personal wounds, was causing problems.

He found himself drawn to patients who shared similar experiences. His intentions were genuine, but his desire to 'fix' others became a dominant driving force in his approach to patient care. Instead of maintaining professional boundaries, Alex became emotionally invested in his patients' outcomes, contacting them out of hours to 'just check up on them', lending them money and buying them food if they were hungry. As time passed, the weight of their patients' struggles and his unresolved wounds became overwhelming, and he decided to give up medical training.

As mentioned earlier, when exploring the Wounded Healer concept, the draw to a caring profession may stem from early, unresolved experiences of illness, including the loss or illness of a parent. When exposed to similar experiences in their work, this can become a compulsion to save, even when it may be futile or overwhelming. While these behaviours may initially seem positive and productive, they can ultimately lead to negative consequences such as burnout, depression and anxiety.

The commonly cited reasons include a love for science, a desire to help people, the various opportunities available, flexibility, job security, familial influence or the desire for financial stability or prestige.

Unconscious motivations can be more complex and manifest differently throughout a doctor's career. Some individuals' personal experiences with illness or trauma may have played an essential role in their decision to pursue medicine. This experience of emotional suffering can provide individuals with a unique perspective and understanding of the patient experience, which can be valuable in health care. This may also inspire individuals to use their own experiences to help others who are going through similar struggles. Sarinda, who gave his account earlier in this handbook, highlights some of these unconscious drivers, including the need to feel a worthy 'return on investment' for his parents, the desire to fix others where a part of self was perceived as broken; and to please and seek validation from others, feeding a desire for a sense of self-worth.

Other unconscious motivations that may lead to a career in medicine include:

- Compensation for a past traumatic experience or loss.
- The desire for control and power over life and death.
- Need for approval and validation from others.
- Desire to please or appease a parent or authority figure.
- Fear of failure or not living up to expectations.
- The feeling of obligation to give back to society or those who have helped.
- The desire for a sense of identity or purpose.

5

Risk of mental illness

Doctors do not work in a vacuum. Their working conditions are influenced by the environment and culture in which they work. Not having enough resources to employ sufficient cover for the absence of colleagues or mechanisms to reduce the intensity of the workload can, if prolonged, negatively impact a doctor's health. This chapter addresses some of these factors.

SOCIO-POLITICAL FACTORS

Socio-political factors can significantly impact a doctor's mental health. For example, funding cuts, staffing shortages and patient demand can increase workload and burnout. Doctors may experience moral distress when asked to provide care that conflicts with their personal or professional values. The global workload crisis in health care is a significant issue, with increasing demands for care and a decrease in the workforce. This crisis has been further exacerbated by the pandemic, which overwhelmed healthcare systems and placed additional strain on healthcare professionals. The staff shortage has made addressing the backlog of patients needing treatment even more challenging.

Efforts to reduce working hours for doctors, particularly junior doctors, have had mixed results. While shorter shifts can help prevent fatigue-related errors, they can also create challenges regarding handover and continuity. Additionally, some studies have suggested that reducing working hours may not necessarily lead to improved patient outcomes, as it may reduce the time doctors spend with each patient.

Major political events can influence the mood of doctors. A study conducted in the United States looked at the impact of macro-level factors, such as national elections, on junior doctors' mental health. The most significant impact was following the 2016 Presidential Election, with women reporting a more significant decline in mood than male doctors.[38]

DOI: 10.1201/9781003391500-5

CULTURE AND PRACTICE

The culture of medicine refers to the shared values within the medical profession. It encompasses many factors influencing behaviour and attitudes and how staff interact with patients and other stakeholders. It reflects the shared values, beliefs and behaviours underpinning doctors' working lives. It comprises the complex interplay between the individual doctor, the system in which they work, their training and the society in which they are immersed. Cultural norms are often unseen, yet powerful and pervasive, and can change, albeit slowly over time, depending on prevailing pressures and through the influence of leaders.

One key aspect of the culture of medicine is the emphasis on professionalism, which includes values such as honesty, integrity and a commitment to the welfare of patients. Professionalism refers to individuals' behaviours, attitudes and qualities in their work or professional roles. It involves adhering to high standards of ethical conduct, demonstrating competence and maintaining a respectful and responsible demeanour. Another essential feature is the emphasis on scientific knowledge and evidence-based practice. Medical professionals are expected to stay current on the latest research and developments in their field and use this knowledge to inform their clinical decision-making.

The culture of medicine also includes certain practices and rituals unique to the profession, such as rites of passage, which mark the transition from student to doctor. These include rituals of separation between the medical and non-medical student, absorbing biomedical knowledge, skills, attitudes, values and so on, and the way of incorporation through the swearing of the Hippocratic Oath, the label of '*Dr.*' and distinctive uniform.

Culture has both visible and invisible, as well as conscious and unconscious, manifestations. For example, the design of clinics, often over-running with patients waiting hours beyond the scheduled appointment time, perpetuates the expectation that a patient's time is less important than the doctor's time, reinforcing the unconscious hierarchy between the two. The culture of medicine also brings with it the tacit agreement that doctors will sacrifice themselves for the service of their patients, which can lead to unhealthy norms and potentially harmful behaviours, such as doctors denying their own needs as if typical vulnerabilities do not apply to them. Ingrained cultural norms can also create problems. For example, the culture of medicine, especially hospital medicine, does not cater for supporting female doctors who often have other caring roles – both for children and elders.

BLAME AND FEAR

Fear is embedded within the culture of medicine

Fear distorts one's perception of reality, causing individuals to view situations through anxiety and insecurity. This can affect people at various levels of responsibility, from employees to managers and leaders. When fear is present, people tend to prioritise their self-interests and concerns, such as job security and reputation. For example, in a work environment, doctors may fear making mistakes or facing negative consequences. This fear can influence their decision-making process as they focus more on protecting their job security and preserving their organisational reputation.

Modern healthcare systems, far from encouraging transparency, often do the opposite, and when an error is made, the first reaction tends to be a need to apportion blame. In his book *Zero*, a former Secretary of Health (England), Jeremy Hunt,[39] writes about the blame culture he has experienced. Hunt describes the covering up of mistakes as 'endemic'. In circumstances where life is lost or serious incidents have been made, there seems to be a tendency for individuals and whole institutions to gloss over the true nature of events leading up to an incident. Hunt concludes that systemic defensiveness is partly a symptom of blame culture, where institutions can enter self-preservation status because of pervasive fear. If fear pervades healthcare culture, repeated mistakes and harm are an inevitability.

Fear is at the heart of the factors contributing to physician mental illness and suicide. Doctors fear losing their professional identity, being cast out of medicine, becoming a patient, being abused and excluded, making mistakes, upsetting seniors and failing to meet patient expectations.

Fear can be helpful; it helps us anticipate danger and take constructive action to mitigate damage. But when working life is built on fear, it becomes unsustainable and affects the individual's mental health.

There are several reasons why a culture of fear and blame is so prevalent in health organisations:

- There is a high risk of legal action against healthcare providers in case of medical errors or adverse outcomes. This can create a culture where individuals are hesitant to admit mistakes or take responsibility for their actions, leading to a fear of litigation.

- Healthcare organisations are often hierarchical, with senior staff having more power and influence than junior staff. This can create a culture where blame is passed down the chain of command, with junior staff members being held responsible for errors resulting from systemic issues or decisions made by senior staff.

- Healthcare organisations may not have transparent processes for reporting and investigating errors or adverse events. This lack of transparency can create a culture where mistakes are covered up rather than used as an opportunity for learning and improvement.

- Healthcare professionals are under significant pressure to perform their duties to the best of their abilities, often in high-stress environments. This pressure can lead to a culture where blame motivates individuals to perform better rather than focusing on systemic issues that may be contributing to errors.

STIGMA

Stigma is a term used to describe specific characteristics or traits that can make an individual appear unacceptable or different in the eyes of the prevailing culture or society. These characteristics can vary depending on cultural norms and values. Stigma often leads to feelings of shame, which is an intense perception of embarrassment or disgrace associated with being marked as different or deviating from societal norms and is a typical emotional response when someone feels stigmatised. When stigma is present, responsibility is often attributed to the individual, suggesting they are responsible for their differences or perceived shortcomings. The guilt and stigma experienced by an individual can result in their exclusion from specific social groups or settings. This exclusion can take various forms, including marginalisation in the workplace.

'**Enacted stigma**' refers to the experiences of marginalisation, discrimination or mistreatment that individuals face due to the stigma attached to their characteristics, leading to feelings of loneliness, loss and sadness for the stigmatised individuals. Enacted stigma at work can create significant challenges for individuals who have experienced illness or other circumstances that require time off. Returning to work after such absences becomes more difficult due to the emotional toll of being stigmatised and marginalised.[40]

Stigma can be rooted in cultural, religious and social beliefs, misconceptions and lack of awareness about mental health. For example, traditional cultural values that emphasise conformity, collective harmony and face-saving can contribute to the reluctance to seek help for mental health issues.

SHAME

The medical culture engenders a loss of personal agency and a diminished sense of competence, which not only adversely affects the well-being of doctors but indirectly impacts the quality of patient care they provide.[41]

Shame is an intrinsic part of the human experience and arises when one's values are questioned. While shame can positively motivate doctors to commit to altruism and ethical conduct, the erosion of autonomy compels doctors to conform to the behaviours of their professional group, often learned through the hidden curriculum or the unspoken code of conduct in medical education.

Within the medical field, shame manifests in various behaviours, including a silent withdrawal from social interactions, a tendency to appease and seek approval and resorting to shaming or blaming others for regaining a sense of power.

BULLYING AND RACISM

Bullying can lead to physical and mental health problems for both victim and perpetrator, decreased productivity and morale among other employees, and a hostile work environment and a high turnover.

Bullying is common and extensively reported, with up to a third of NHS staff saying they had experienced bullying in the past year. Doctors from Black and Asian backgrounds were more likely to report bullying than White doctors, and women were more likely to report bullying than men.

Bullying in the workplace can be challenging to define, as there is no explicit agreement on what constitutes adult bullying. Most definitions consist of a few key elements: Firstly, the effect on the victim rather than the intention of the bully determines if bullying has occurred, making it subject to variations in personal perception; there must have been a negative impact on the victim; and finally, the behaviour must be persistent over time.

Bullying is persistent behaviour against an individual that is intimidating, degrading, offensive or malicious and undermines the confidence and self-esteem of the recipient. Harassment is unwanted behaviour due to age, sex, race, disability, religion, sexuality, or any personal characteristic of the individual. It may be persistent or an isolated incident.

Five types of workplace bullying have been identified:

1. **Isolation:** Ignoring, preventing someone from having access to opportunities, and having essential information withheld that might hinder their ability to work.
2. **Threat to personal standing:** Spreading rumours, name-calling, gossiping.
3. **Threat to professional status:** Humiliation, accusations regarding poor work and lack of effort, favouring colleagues with career progression.
4. **Destabilisation:** Failure to give credit when due, shifting goalposts, repeated reminders of errors and being given meaningless, time-consuming tasks.
5. **Enforced overwork:** Impossible deadlines and excessive pressure to produce work.

Bullying can also include microaggression

Microaggressions are subtle, often unintentional, everyday actions or comments that communicate derogatory or harmful messages to individuals from marginalised groups. These verbal, non-verbal or environmental actions often reflect deep-seated biases or stereotypes. Microaggressions can contribute to an unwelcoming, hostile or discriminatory environment and can have a cumulative impact on the mental and emotional well-being of individuals who experience them.

In the medical space, microaggressions can manifest in various ways and impact patients and healthcare professionals. Here are some examples of microaggressions in the medical context:

1. **Assumption of language proficiency:** Making the assumption that a healthcare professional from a minority ethnic or linguistic group does not speak or understand the dominant language well, even if they do. For instance, speaking loudly and slowly to a patient with an accent, assuming they need help understanding complex medical terminology.

2. **Mispronouncing names:** Consistently mispronouncing or changing the names of patients or colleagues with non-Western or unfamiliar names, which can be perceived as a lack of respect or disregard for their identity.

3. **Ignoring concerns:** Dismissing or ignoring a patient's concerns or symptoms, attributing them to psychological factors or stress solely based on their identity, gender, or race.

Microaggressions can often be subtle and unintentional, but their impact can be significant. Raising awareness about these issues, educating healthcare professionals about cultural competence and promoting open dialogue can help reduce microaggressions and create a more inclusive and equitable healthcare environment.

INDUSTRIALISATION OF CARE

Peter had been practising medicine for over three decades and had always been deeply passionate about patient care. His hospital had recently implemented new productivity metrics and streamlined processes, shifting the focus from patient-centred care to meeting strict targets and maximising throughput. Doctors were required to see increasing numbers of patients within limited time frames, leaving little room for meaningful connections and personalised care. Peter felt overwhelmed by the constant pressure to meet these new targets. He rushed through patient visits, never feeling he had enough time to address complex medical conditions or the patient's emotional needs. The emphasis on efficiency left him feeling disconnected and joyless from the job he once loved. In addition to the increased workload, Peter faced mounting administrative tasks, which took away time he could have spent providing quality care. He also noticed a shift in the power dynamics within the hospital. Administrators influenced medical decision-making, often prioritising financial considerations over patient well-being. Peter felt frustrated and disempowered, witnessing cases where necessary treatments were denied or delayed due to cost constraints. The cumulative effect of these changes on Peter's mental well-being was significant. He experienced increased stress, anxiety and a

sense of moral distress. Peter wasn't alone. Many colleagues shared similar senti-
ments, expressing burnout, emotional exhaustion and a loss of purpose.

Peter has experienced the industrialisation of health care, which refers to trans-
forming the delivery and practice into a system that mirrors industrial processes
and principles[42] and involves applying efficiency-driven models, standardisa-
tion and cost-cutting measures to healthcare settings, often aiming to maximise
productivity and reduce costs. Various factors, including technological advancements, the influence of Managed Care Organisations in America and Foundation
Trusts in NHS and the shift towards evidence-based medicine, have encouraged
this move. It has led to significant changes in healthcare practices, organisational
structures, doctor–patient relationships and the erosion of traditional values and
professionalism.

It is important to note that while the 'industrialisation' of medicine has led to
advancements and improvements in many aspects of health care, there are ongoing debates about its potential drawbacks, particularly related to patient-centred
care, the doctor–patient relationship and the potential for health care to become
overly mechanistic or profit-driven. Finding a balance between efficiency and
personalised care is essential in this evolving landscape.

THE WORKPLACE

Medicine is a challenging taskmaster. It is more than just the long hours or the
years of gruelling training. It is also the weight of responsibility that comes with
the job. The doctor oversees people's health, happiness and even their lives. The
demands are endless, and one is expected to be an expert in everything from
medicine to management. A doctor will face many challenges affecting their
mental, emotional and physical well-being. They witness other people's suffering,
despair and pain daily, and it can be hard not to let it affect this impact on one's
mental state. They are constantly under pressure to perform, often without the
support or resources to succeed. It is hardly surprising, therefore, that doctors are
at risk of mental illness and that work is a significant contributor.

Several factors within the medical workplace can contribute to the mental health
challenges faced by doctors:

1. **High workload and long hours:** Dealing with increasing numbers of patients,
   many with complex conditions and long shifts due to staff shortages.

2. **Emotional stress:** Dealing with serious illnesses, life-and-death decisions
   and patient suffering can affect doctors' emotional well-being. The constant
   exposure to emotional and distressing situations can lead to compassion
   fatigue and emotional exhaustion.

3. **High expectations and perfectionism:** Doctors may feel immense pressure
   to excel and fear making mistakes, contributing to anxiety and self-criticism.

4. **Lack of control:** Doctors might face situations where they have limited control over patient outcomes due to the complex nature of medical conditions and treatment. This lack of control can lead to frustration and stress.

5. **Administrative burden:** The increasing administrative burden takes time from patient care and can contribute to stress and burnout.

6. **Workplace bullying and harassment:** Workplace bullying, harassment and mistreatment can negatively impact mental health and contribute to a hostile work environment.

7. **The stigma around mental health:** There is often a stigma associated with mental health issues in the medical profession. Doctors might fear seeking help for mental health concerns could jeopardise their careers or reputations.

8. **Isolation and lack of support:** Doctors may experience feelings of isolation due to the nature of their work and the challenges they face. A lack of peer and supervisor support can exacerbate stress and loneliness.

9. **Pressure to perform:** The pressure to meet performance targets, academic expectations and patient satisfaction can lead to constant stress and a fear of not meeting professional standards.

10. **Career uncertainty:** Doctors face a competitive environment for training posts and research opportunities, leading to career uncertainty and anxiety about prospects.

11. **Work-life imbalance:** The demanding nature of medical careers can make it challenging for doctors to maintain a healthy work-life balance, impacting their overall well-being.

12. **Limited time for self-care:** The demanding work schedules often leave doctors with limited time to engage in self-care activities that promote mental and physical well-being.

SLEEP DISTURBANCE

Sleep is an integral component of a healthy lifestyle, with humans biologically hard-wired to be active and alert in the daytime and sleepy at night. Most adults require 7.5–8.5 hours of sleep per night, and deficits in cognitive performance can ensue when acutely or chronically sleep-deprived.[43] To balance this, many people can function on less sleep, and it is probably the function of the quality rather than quantity of sleep that is important.

Healthcare professionals often work antisocial hours and night shifts. This affects not just mental well-being, with chronic sleep deprivation contributing to burn-out, but also performance, with diagnostic errors more common in doctors working long hours or shifts.[44] Furthermore, healthcare professionals' burnout and sleep deprivation have been associated with reduced empathy and cognitive functioning.[45] This highlights the downward spiral of worsening mental well-being that lack of sleep can lead to.

Beyond deteriorating cognitive functions, sleep deprivation and shift work sleep disorder can affect physical health too, with cardiovascular disease, obesity, type 2 diabetes and increased cancer risk associated with a lack of sleep.[46] A significant challenge for shift-working healthcare professionals is sleep short-changing, as daytime sleep is not of equivalent quality or as restorative as sleeping at night.

The Royal College of Physicians has published helpful guidance for junior doctors called '*Working the night shift: preparation, survival and recovery*', which is freely available online at:

• *https://shop.rcplondon.ac.uk/products/working-the-night-shift-preparation-survival-and-recovery?variant=6334287429.*

Shift work, particularly night shifts, can present various challenges for doctors, including:

• **Sleep deprivation:** Working irregular hours can disrupt a person's natural sleep–wake cycle and lead to sleep deprivation, impacting mental and physical health.

• **Fatigue:** Chronic sleep deprivation can lead to chronic fatigue, affecting performance and increasing the risk of errors and accidents.

• **Social and family disruption:** Shift work can disrupt personal relationships, social life and family life, as one's schedule may not align with others.

• **Poor eating habits:** Shift work can lead to poor eating habits, as one may need access to healthy food options or help to eat regularly.

• **Stress:** The demands of shift work and the pressure of providing medical care can increase stress levels and lead to burnout.

• **Health problems:** Chronic shift work has been linked to several health problems, including cardiovascular disease, digestive problems and mental health issues such as depression and anxiety.

WORKLOAD AND INTENSITY OF WORK

Henry struggled to open the surgery door, not because it was physically heavy but because he felt emotionally exhausted. It was still only 7 a.m. – a full hour before the patients would flood in, yet someone was already waiting behind the front door as he let himself through the back door. He recognised the patient as she had been coming to see him with various complaints for years. No matter what he did, she always complained about one thing or another. He couldn't help her anymore; he doubted he could help anyone. Henry had to come earlier and leave later each evening to finish the work. His wife was beginning to accuse him of having an affair – he laughed, if only that were the case. He went to work tired and had difficulty sleeping. He resented his wife gently snoring next to him as he tossed and turned all night, waking early each morning un-refreshed and hung over from the little alcohol he had the previous evening to help him get off to sleep.

His consulting room had remained unchanged for the years. He moved into it soon after the senior partner retired. The space once had a piano – courtesy of his retired partner, who used to play it during breaks and occasionally let patients play to help them relax. It felt like his transitional object – a link to the idealised glory days of the practice, when it was thriving and fully staffed, an abundance of health professionals wandering in and out each day, all excited about the developments in the surgery and local area, growth and innovation seemed to be the buzz words, and life felt good. He was younger then, just starting in general practice, and his wife was expecting their first child. Last year, they failed to recruit a partner, and he had unfilled vacancies in most roles. He knew that once surgery opened and the phones were switched over, there would be many patients, endless calls, paperwork and demands from others. Last week, he had 300 letters from the local hospital – almost all ending with 'GP to do'. He thought about the meeting with his partners that evening. He had been carrying around a resignation letter for a few weeks and felt he would give it to them this evening. He thought that he couldn't go on anymore. Henry began to cry.

It seems evident that work intensity and intolerable workloads contribute to mental illness. Still, it is worth saying, as often it is a doctor's 'lack of resilience' rather than the conditions they work in which is blamed for their mental illness. Doctors are some of the most resilient members of the workforce. They are used to working long hours, often without a break. They can go from one traumatic experience to another and function well in a crisis. They can 'bounce back' and learn from negative (and positive) experiences.

But as with any object, given enough environmental pressure, they have their breaking point beyond which they can go no further. It is the intensity of the work, which includes factors such as high stress, long working hours and high-pressure decision-making, which contributes to mental illness by increasing feelings of burnout, anxiety and depression.

Ignoring environmental (work-related) factors in the pathogenesis of mental illness and instead focusing on the individual diverts attention from the structural and organisational factors within the healthcare system that contribute to stress, burnout and mental health issues among healthcare professionals. Focusing solely on resilience implies that doctors should be able to handle any challenges without considering whether the system contributes to their difficulties.

It is difficult to say which is worse, the intensity of work or the workload, as both factors can significantly impact physician well-being and contribute to mental illness. Both high power and high workload can lead to stress, burnout and a reduced sense of well-being.

ORGANISATION, RESILIENCE AND WORKING PRACTICES

Doctors have always worked close to death, distress and disability and are used to long, unsocial hours and hard work. This has not changed, though the working environment has changed over the last decade, and this might be the barrier to developing resilience and mental health robustness. How medicine is organised and the rise in blame, bullying and retribution negates the development of resilience. Paradoxically, shorter working hours are also a barrier to developing resilience. The 48-hour working time directive means doctors work shifts that fracture teamwork – essential to creating the relationships that build support, feedback and strength for training grade doctors. Just as continuity of care for patients is valued, so is it amongst those who care for them, continuity in terms of looking after their patients from admission to discharge, but also continuity of space (wards, hospitals, homes) and colleagues (peers, trainers, nurses); are mainly absent in many of these areas.

Michael West, an organisational psychologist, was commissioned by the General Medical Council (GMC) to review factors within the workplace impacting the mental health of medical students and doctors in training.[47]

The three areas most pertinent to well-being and related to the workplace were as follows:

- **Autonomy:** Control over work life and working consistently according to one's values.

- **Belonging:** Connection to, caring for by and caring for others in the workplace, generated value, respect and support.

- **Competence:** Delivering a valued outcome effectively, such as high-quality, compassionate care.

The report 'Caring for Doctors, Caring for Patients',[47] commented that '*the role of doctors in training seems perversely designed to prevent the fulfilment of all three needs*' (p. 71) in particular, that trainee doctors are particularly vulnerable to workplace stressors; there is a disproportionate level of service provision compared to the time allocated for training and education; the rigidity of the movement is counter-intuitive to development; and this all impacts on the ability to pass several exams, leading to differential attainments and financial pressures especially if retaking assessments.

6

The doctor and their speciality

SPECIALITY

Comparing mental morbidity between different medical specialities is challenging due to several factors. Variables, such as the location of work, type of hospital or community setting, staffing ratios and work intensity, can significantly influence mental health outcomes, making it difficult to attribute differences solely to the speciality. Additionally, defining what constitutes a speciality is complex. For example, even within a narrower speciality such as neurology, there can be work, environment, and cultural variations between subspecialties such as neurology and neurophysiology. Similarly, cardiology can be further subdivided into divisions such as interventional imaging or heart failure, each with its unique working patterns and practice. As such, only a few of the larger high-level specialities are discussed below, where meaningful interpretations of the data and comments can be made.

GENERAL PRACTITIONERS

General practice across the world is in crisis. Workload has increased substantially in recent years and has yet to be matched by growth in either funding or workforce.

Pressures on general practice are compounded by the work becoming more complex and intense. This is mainly due to the ageing population, increasing numbers of people with long term conditions, initiatives to move care from hospitals to the community and rising public expectations. Surveys show that general practitioners (GPs) in the NHS report finding their job more stressful than their counterparts in other countries.

Fewer GPs are choosing to undertake full-time clinical work, with more opting for portfolio careers or working part-time. This is true for both male and female GPs. This continues a long-term trend in which fewer doctors aspire to become partners in their practices.

In the UK NHS, around three-quarters of healthcare contacts take place with a GP, and it is often the first port of call for patients with acute conditions. It is also where most of the care of patients with long-term conditions takes place.

UK general practice faces significant problems maintaining the GP workforce, with GP shortages and a potential risk to patient care.

A near quadrupling of unfilled GP posts since 2010 and an overall reduction in GPs means that those working carry an ever-increasing work burden. Compounded with the shortage in the workforce is the ageing GP population, with more than a third of GPs over the age of 50 years.

Matthew wanted to be a GP since medical school, influenced by his science teacher, who persuaded him to try medicine. In recent years, he felt he was drowning in an overwhelming workload. The days he seemed to blur together as he rushed from one patient to another, with barely a moment to catch his breath. The waiting room overflowed with people seeking his care, their concerns piling up like an insurmountable mountain.

Every day, he felt an increasing sense of helplessness. The demands on his time and attention left little room for self-care, reflection, or even essential rest. The endless stream of paperwork, the constant need to keep up with medical advancements, and the pressure to provide accurate diagnoses and effective treatments pushed him to the edge. At night, he experienced sleepless battles, restless with thoughts plagued by the fear of missing critical details or making mistakes that could have serious consequences for his patients. The joy and enthusiasm that once fuelled his passion for medicine began to flicker, overshadowed by a cloud of fatigue and despair. His personal life was suffering as well. He became withdrawn from his loved ones, unable to engage in conversations or find solace in their company entirely. He felt isolated as if his struggles were invisible to those around him.

Given their position at the 'front door' of the health system, GPs probably bear a disproportionate workload burden against diminishing resources. It is hardly surprising; therefore, they often present with mental distress and burnout.

PSYCHIATRISTS

Jane, a psychiatrist in a community placement, was proud that she offered hope to individuals struggling with mental health issues, offering them kindness, understanding and guidance. However, she entered the department with a sense of emptiness. The patients, each presenting unique issues, had begun eroding the walls she had erected to protect her sanity. Her days became a blur of back-to-back sessions, the hours blending as she listened to stories of pain, trauma, and anguish. The suffering of her patients stayed with her even as she left to go home, leaving her feeling drained and discouraged. She could no longer separate her patients' pain from her own, as if their struggles had become an inescapable part of her existence. She lay awake at night, consumed by the echoes of her patients' stories. The boundaries between her personal and professional life blurred. The once clear distinction between empathy and her emotional well-being became muddied, and she questioned if she could continue down this path. The burnout that had slowly been festering within her was manifesting in her interactions with her patients, leaving her feeling even more guilty and inadequate.

Psychiatrists are reported to have higher rates of mental illness than most other doctors, with high levels of stress, job dissatisfaction, depression and burnout. This might be for several reasons. These include factors such as exposure to patient violence and suicide, limited resources, crowded inpatient wards, changing culture in mental health services, high work demands, poorly defined roles of consultants, responsibility without authority, inability to effect systemic change, the conflict between responsibility towards employers *versus* towards the patients, and isolation.

Concerning the work itself, as Jane demonstrates, the courageous actions of psychiatrists are mainly invisible. It takes enormous mental strength to remain focused when listening to the psychic pain of patients, day in and day out. This intense doctor–patient relationship is complex and unpredictable. Patients evoke emotions such as the need to be rescued and a sense of failure and frustration when they cannot and when their illness does not respond to treatment. This forms part of the emotional work which all doctors must confront. However, the chronicity and fluctuating nature of their patients' illnesses can be particularly challenging for psychiatrists.

Whilst blame seems to be inherent in the whole health system, for psychiatrists, this is particularly acute as they are held responsible when a patient with mental illness takes their own life or kills or harms another. Psychiatrists must undertake the difficult, if not impossible, task of assigning risk status to a patient before discharge and predicting future behaviour. Most psychiatrists experience the death of a patient by suicide at least once in their career, which can have profound and long-term effects on their personal, psychological and professional lives.[48]

Those who go into the mental health field (counsellors, psychiatrists, psychotherapists) might be more likely to have a history of mental health problems themselves, entering the area as a vicarious desire to understand their difficulties or in the hope of repairing past traumas.

There is evidence that despite higher rates of mental illness, psychiatrists are more reluctant to attend treatment, even when these services offer confidential care. Stigma to mental illness is not an abstract issue for this speciality group. They see their patients exposed to it daily. When mentally unwell themselves, they are on the receiving end, leading to deep-seated shame and guilt. Self-stigmatisation is not uncommon. It is also challenging for a psychiatrist to receive confidential help, as with GPs, if they work and live in the same area.

SURGEONS

Examining research findings based on surveys and in numbers attending treatment services, it appears that surgeons have a lower mental illness rate than other doctors. This might be due to several reasons.

A lower presentation rate could be due to surgeons having more protective factors (e.g., better resilience to cope with occupational stress). There might be some validity in this, as those who cannot cope with the pressure and competitiveness of a surgical career may fall along the way, leaving only the fittest to survive. Surgeons might be protected by their close working relationships with others, allowing for sharing of distress, successes and general support. An aura of authority surrounds surgeons. This authority is generally unquestioned, and confidence seen externally might be reflected internally.

An alternative explanation is that they are more reluctant to seek help than their non-surgical peers. There is some evidence for this. There is some validation in this, as surveys show high levels of suicidal ideation (especially in older surgeons), significant levels of distress, anxiety and burnout, yet lower levels of presentation to treatment services.

It should not be surprising that surgeons might have high rates of mental illness, given their long, unpredictable hours and high-stress work. All doctors have their unwritten group norms developed over generations. For surgeons, these include working long hours (sometimes when not even rostered to do so), meeting multiple deadlines, rarely complaining, and keeping emotions or personal problems away from the workspace. They also have some of the most extended medical training and make substantial personal sacrifices to achieve their chosen profession. Surgeons must consistently perform well, always under the spotlight of others (at the very least, scrub nurses and anaesthetists). They also need to appear competent, irrespective of their internal demons. In the operating theatre, the surgeon must take control and rescue the situation when the going gets tough. Even when off-duty, surgeons may ruminate over a complex forthcoming operation or worry about the patient in intensive care; there are other contributing factors in the development of mental illness among surgeons. Patients are at their most vulnerable when they see a surgeon, whether unconscious on the operating table or lying on their hospital bed in anticipation of reassurances, pre- or post-operative. Patients trust surgeons. They relinquish all authority and power to them. They become helpless. The surgeon's job requires constantly containing others' fears of death. This places a heavy toll on the individual doctor. The expectations placed on surgeons might make it harder to accept vulnerability and present for care when needed. Instead, they must project the image of being tough and resilient.

Surgeons have low rates of substance misuse. Close working relationships, with every move witnessed, lengthy and unpredictable hours of work, frequent on-call shifts and out-of-hours work, would make it difficult to disguise an alcohol or drug problem.

ANAESTHETISTS

Easy access to intravenous opioids and anaesthetic agents, including inhalation gases, places anaesthetists at particular risk of addiction and death due to drug overdose. Estimating the true prevalence of substance misuse disorder is difficult as even in surveys promising confidentiality, and there is a reluctance to admit to a problem that could result in criminal and professional sanctions. Where studies have been done, the risk for anaesthetists is reported to be nearly three times that of other doctors.[49]

Unfortunately, the first indication that an anaesthetist has a problem might be death from accidental or deliberate overdose. **Suicide is reported to be the cause of death in approximately 6%–10% of anaesthetists, and the risk of a drug-related death is nearly three times that of a general physician.**[49]

Nearly 40% of anaesthetists working in the UK and Ireland have had first-hand experience of an anaesthetic colleague who has died by their hand (either accidental or deliberate). This shows death's impact and reach on those in the same speciality. Most of these deaths involved anaesthetic agents.[50]

PAEDIATRICIANS

Safeguarding issues apart (where parents' wishes might not always be aligned with those of children and doctors), paediatricians have traditionally enjoyed a close working relationship with children and families, which has been a positively reinforcing factor for those working in the field. A further attraction has been the most transformative act of improving children's health speedily. However, advances in technology and medicine mean that this is changing. As more children survive with medically complex conditions, paediatric wards are no longer filled with patients who bounce back to health within 24 hours; instead, beds are occupied by children with multiple healthcare needs, disability and life-limiting illnesses. The fragmented health, education and social care systems often fail to serve these children and their families well. Inadequate resources, difficulty managing complexity and uncertainty, and a mismatch between expectations and what is deliverable add to this inability to deliver the best care. As a result, parents are often distressed, frustrated and exhausted. Paediatricians report high stress levels just doing a routine ward round in the face of this tension.

VULNERABLE GROUPS

Even within the cohort of doctors, some groups will be more vulnerable due to inherent stereotyping, stigma and cultural issues. One of the most isolating positions is when someone is seemingly part of the 'group' but does not feel they are indeed a part of it.

INTERNATIONAL MEDICAL GRADUATES (IMGs)

An **international medical graduate (IMG)** is a medical doctor who has completed their medical education and training in a country other than where they intend to practise medicine. The term is often used in countries where medical training and licensing requirements vary, and foreign-trained doctors must undergo additional steps to practise medicine within their borders.

Below is a personal account written by a doctor from overseas who went to work in the NHS.

Two years ago, I arrived in Britain on the overseas doctors' training scheme in psychiatry. This was my first trip to a foreign country. I came with little money and no friends or relatives in Britain. For someone who has always been one of us, it is impossible to imagine the feeling of being the other that engulfs you soon after arrival in a new country. The deafening silence of the countryside, the palpable discomfort at meeting a stranger's gaze, astonishment at everyone's attempts to hide behind a newspaper in the London Tube, inability to react to the smile of a stranger that never quite reaches the eyes, and the early awareness of racial stereotypes are all disconcerting experiences. You are torn between the need for human contact and a greater need to hide. For most people, a summation of discrete experiences crystallises into this feeling of otherness.[51]

The relationship between the UK healthcare system and IMGs is a long-standing one that predates the establishment of the NHS. IMGs have added diversity to the NHS and allowed it to grow and develop by bringing in new perspectives and helping to boost specialities with recruitment gaps.

Many doctors on the General Medical Council (GMC) register of licenced practitioners are IMGs, and their numbers are growing. There are also increasing numbers of students born in the UK and with British nationality choosing to train overseas. Whilst these doctors do not suffer as many problems as those IMGs with non-UK born, they still experience discrimination and other issues described below.

IMGs have always faced difficulties moving to a new country – getting used to an unfamiliar healthcare system, adjusting to cultural changes and building a new home. They are often in jobs deemed more challenging, under-resourced and posts in more deprived areas. They frequently work non-training positions and find it more challenging to get onto training schemes, perhaps due to the difficulties of demonstrating competencies without the formal documentation the UK training system provides.[52]

Some of the common problems IMGs face include the following:

- Getting their medical qualifications and experience recognised in their new country can lead to delays in getting licensed to practise medicine.

- Language difficulties can impact being able to communicate effectively with patients and colleagues.

- Adapting to their new country's cultural norms and customs can affect their work performance and relationships with others.

- Prejudice or discrimination from colleagues or patients based on their country of origin or accent.

- Limited job opportunities, particularly in highly competitive speciality fields, are due to a perceived lack of experience or recognition of their qualifications.

- Required to take licensing exams to practice medicine, which can be challenging and time-consuming.

- Building a professional network can impact their career advancement and job prospects.

A vicious cycle ensues, where inequalities impact mental well-being, affecting clinical performance and leading to work difficulties and psychological distress.

Support of IMGs

1. British International Doctors Association (BIDA) *http://www.bidaonline.co.uk/*

2. British Association of Doctors of Indian Origin (BAPIO) *https://www.bapio.co.uk*

3. Burmese Doctors and Dentists Association UK (BDDAUK) *http://www.bdauk.org*

4. British Islamic Medical Association (BIMA) *http://www.britishima.org*

5. British Iranian Medical Association *http://www.bima-uk.com*

6. Muslim Doctors Association *http://www.muslimdoctors.org*

7. Sri Lankan Medical and Dental Association in the UK (SMDA) *http://www.srilankan-mda.org.uk/*

8. Greek Medical Association UK *http://www.greekmeds.co.uk/*

9. Italian Medical Society of Great Britain *http://www.imsogb.org*

10. Medical Association of Nigerians across Great Britain (MANSAG) *http://www.mansag.org/*

11. Nepalese Doctors Association UK (NDAUK) *http://www.ndauk.org.uk*

12. Jewish Medical Association *http://jewishmedicalassociationuk.org/about-jma*

13. BMA – *Are you new to working in the UK*
    https://www.bma.org.uk/advice/work-life-support/life-and-work-in-the-uk/
    guide-for-doctors-new-to-the-uk

14. Health Careers – *information for overseas doctors*
    https://www.healthcareers.nhs.uk/i-am/outside-uk/information-overseas-doctors

15. *https://uima.org.uk/For Iraqi doctors*

FEMALE DOCTORS

Clare had always dreamed of becoming a paediatric surgeon. From a young age, she was fascinated by the intricacies of the human body and dreamt of the opportunity to save children through her skilled hands. She entered medical school and specialised early in her chosen career. She climbed the ranks of her profession, earning recognition for her exceptional surgical skills. She became known for her focus, precision, and ability to handle even the most complex cases with grace and composure. The operating room was her sanctuary, where she felt a sense of purpose and fulfilment like no other.

However, as her career progressed, she realised that her desire to succeed had come at a cost. The sacrifices she had made along the way began to weigh heavily on her. Despite her success in the professional realm, there was an empty void in her personal life. She had dedicated herself entirely to her career, often working long hours, sacrificing weekends and holidays, and putting her patients' needs above hers. She postponed starting a family, believing she could make up for it once she had achieved her professional goals. But as the years passed, she yearned for the joys of motherhood, the warmth of a loving partner and the support of friends who truly understood her.

One evening, as she stood alone in the quiet hallway outside the operating room, exhaustion etched on her face, she realised the effort her choices had taken. Once steady and unwavering, her hands now trembled with fatigue and regret. The realisation hit her: She had sacrificed too much. She began to question whether her pursuit of perfection had been worth her sacrifices.

Research has shown a higher prevalence of female doctors presenting with mental health problems when compared to their male counterparts. This is across the range of severity from psychological distress and mental illness to suicidal ideation, attempts at suicide and completed suicide.[53,54] Young female doctors report more significant stress at work and the compounding challenges of career, family, and significant life events that may occur when life goals are re-assessed, especially when tensions between family and career arise. Taking maternity leave may create anxiety over a pause in training or leaving colleagues on busy rotas, possibly due to a history of inadequate rota cover. Pregnant mothers may find themselves working demanding shifts and find little in the way of support when organising their leave, as well as returning from it. For those women who have family responsibilities, they have the additional demands of the 'second shift' – caring and nurturing their patients during the day, followed by their families in the evening and at night.

The inevitable demands of juggling family life and maternity leave, menopausal symptoms alongside professional responsibilities can cause difficulties for women doctors.

It can be a struggle for junior trainees to manage family demands alongside overnight on-call shifts and exams.

Female doctors suffer discrimination and are overlooked for promotion (in favour of a male counterpart), and 90% of female doctors are victims of sexual harassment in the workplace from staff and patients.[55]

Women are also more likely to be subject to age bias when they are younger because they're thought to be too young to know what they are doing. Yet, when older, they are told they are too old to keep up with current medical changes.

7

Factors influencing seeking help

All doctors will become patients at some point; it is impossible to avoid this. They are as susceptible as the general population to mental and physical illness. They become pregnant, require routine immunisations, have accidents, and have traumatic life events. They are also more likely to develop mental illness. Yet, there are many barriers to presentation, summarised below and which will be looked at in more detail in this chapter, see Table 7.1

Table 7.1 Barriers to seeking help over mental illness	
Area	**Summary of barriers to help for mental health problems**
Work related	• Concerns about career if one admits mental ill health • Concerns about confidentiality • Concerns that disclosure of mental illness might require employment or regulatory involvement which could lead to investigations or curtailment of work
Psychological	• Feelings of shame and embarrassment • Pressure for doctors to appear healthy • Doctors may see illness as a mark of failure • The stigma associated with mental illness • Like anyone else, doctors can deny or minimise their struggles, attributing them to stress or fatigue rather than a genuine problem
Structural	• Lack of confidential services • Lack of specialist skilled staff able to manage fellow health professionals. Frequent changes of address make it difficult to build up a sustaining relationship with a GP or mental health service • Inconsistent access to occupational health services • Challenge to find time in busy schedules and reluctance to burden other doctors' time and workload • Unsupportive environment at work to foster self-care • Lack of information of where to turn to for help
Other	• Doctors might hesitate to seek help from their colleagues, fearing they will receive a different quality of care than they would offer their patients

DOI: 10.1201/9781003391500-7

Some essential and recurrent themes emerge in the following sections.

FEAR OF LACK OF CONFIDENTIALITY

Perhaps the most significant barrier to doctors seeking help is the fear of losing confidentiality, and their problems will be disclosed beyond the consulting room. This might not be due to the treating doctor breaching confidentiality, but finding a confidential space to seek help is hard. Medicine is a small world, and it does not take long for two doctors who have never met each other to find they have friends or colleagues in common. Now factor in a doctor who might live in the same area as they work. Their local hospital is also where they work or where all their neighbouring practices have the same clinical network. This makes it very difficult to consult with someone you don't know personally or professionally (or one's spouse doesn't). At a pinch, this might be acceptable if the reason for needing consulting is not for a sensitive issue. However, if the cause is mental illness or a more personal problem, it might be challenging to discuss with close friends or colleagues. Perhaps the most extreme example of the inability to obtain a confidential space was that of a psychiatrist, who, having attended his own GP for help with depression, found a few weeks later at his referral management multidisciplinary team meeting that he had been referred to himself. The fear of breach of confidentiality also relates to the knowledge of one's illness being relayed beyond the privacy field[56] of the consulting room to workplace supervisors, medical directors, appraisers, employers etc. Once a mental illness has been disclosed, it is not uncommon for many individuals, each with a different 'professional hat', to become involved when a doctor becomes sick. This is especially so for junior-grade doctors.

ADAPTING TO THE PATIENT ROLE

In her book *Illness as Metaphor*, Susan Sontag describes an illness as

> ... is the night-side of life, more onerous citizenship. All born hold dual citizenship in the kingdom of the well and the kingdom of the sick. Although we all prefer to use only the good passport, sooner or later, each of us is obliged, at least for a spell, to identify ourselves as citizens of that other place.[56]

Doctors perhaps find it most challenging to hold dual nationality – that of a patient and that of the healer.

There is an adage that *doctors make bad patients*. And overall, as this book has described, they do. Even once they attend, and in the safety of a consulting room, doctors often start the consultation with a variation on '*I am so sorry to trouble you, sorry to be wasting your time*'.

However, when doctors do present for help, each has their own story of pain and distress, and all have good reasons to seek help. Many have reached the end of their ability to self-sacrifice and to care, and their professional, personal and social lives are often in tatters. They have waited too long to seek help, and when adversity strikes, they work harder, believing that their problems will magically disappear.

Amongst doctors, including those unwell, there can be a thinly veiled criticism of the chronically ill or dependent, the patient who won't '*just help themselves*'. Certain patients quickly become labelled difficult or 'heartsink', and there is an inherent invalidation of their suffering in this.[57] This association between vulnerability and failure can become fixed in the doctor's mind and make admitting vulnerability in oneself even more difficult.

Doctors are trained to place patients' needs above their own, neglecting themselves and gaining satisfaction or praise. This can play into their internal sense and social expectation that they will not require the same levels of care and attention to maintain wellness as they expect their patients to receive.

An uncomfortable stereotype widely held by the public is that doctors are arrogant. As with many stereotypes, there will be doctors who fit in and doctors who certainly do not. However, doctors are often told that they are high achievers – successful, influential and respected members of society. This is bound to have an inflating effect. When this person then needs to 'cross over' to the role of patient, it can feel demeaning and shameful.[40] Becoming unwell and needing to accept a state of vulnerability can be described psychoanalytically as a narcissistic wound, triggering defensive mechanisms such as denial, omnipotence and other ego-defences discussed earlier in this book. Fear of lack of privacy can, on the one hand, be a realistic concern but, on the other, could be seen as a paranoid ego-defence. The defence, expressed as the fear that their information will be leaked or fall into the wrong hands, protects the sense of importance from intrusion.

Over the years, many doctors have written about their experiences of becoming patients and how this has influenced their practice. These personal accounts help ground doctors and demystify the impact of becoming a patient.

Kay McCall,[22] for example, a GP who suffered from bipolar disorder, wrote in 2001,[58]

> *I've become sensitive to what other doctors make when managing me, and I have translated those mistakes into corrections in managing people with depression. The point of this article is to share these with you.*

Kate Granger,[23] who died from metastatic sarcoma, started the '#hellomynameis' campaign encouraging healthcare staff to introduce themselves to patients and wrote a book,

> *to be better able to understand exactly what being the patient is really like and how their behaviours, no matter how small can impact massively on the people they look after.*

The GP and writer Jonathon Tomlinson has examined the themes which emerge from first-person testimonies,[59] and the experience doctors have crossed the divide into parenthood. Tomlinson identifies four common themes which doctors experience. They are the loss of professional identity, shame and stigma, the need to be seen as a person and poor standards of care.

That illness shatters a doctor's professional identity was identified through the work of Alex Wessely, who, as part of his anthropology dissertation, tried to understand why doctors made good addicts and bad patients (quoting the title of his thesis). They become 'good addicts' because they can work despite severe impairment and, in doing so, deny or disavow any vulnerability or need to seek help. They saw themselves as invincible.[60] In a paper published in the *British Medical Journal*, he wrote,[61]

> The nature of doctors' training results in a deep-rooted sense of being special and the institutionalisation of their professional identity, with the creation of a medical self that ... allows doctors to do their job effectively when they must deal with stressful and long hours and provides the veneer of invincibility to live and work in such proximity with sickness. These characteristics, however, also distort doctors' ability to seek help and adopt the role of the patient. For example, when accompanying a relative or friend to the hospital, doctors often find it hard to relinquish their professional role and be the concerned lay 'other.' Abandoning their medical self is challenging, even in the short term. This dissonance might also explain why doctors can sacrifice their personal, social, financial, and often spiritual lives at work, remaining there long beyond what would be considered safe for themselves or their patients.

Shame, a subject already discussed in this handbook, is a significant feature in the reluctance to become a patient. Patienthood is associated (in the minds of doctors) with loss of status, identity and failure to comply with the unwritten rule, '*It is patients who are unwell, not doctors*'.

When sick, healthcare professionals find it challenging to take time off work ('*presenteeism*'). One study shows that more than a third of doctors and nurses go to work despite feeling they should have taken sick leave, whereas only a quarter took time off work for health reasons. Doctors worry about the disapproval of their medical colleagues and must deal with their feelings of guilt and shame.[41]

There is little research to guide how doctors on both sides of the fence should behave when unwell or consulting with a sick colleague. The GMC and British Medical Association (BMA) do provide some guidance. They stress that the underlying principle is that a doctor's first concern is the patient and doctors who happen to be patients are entitled to the same high standards of care.

Guidance from the GMC[62] and BMA[63] on how doctors should manage their health:

- Doctors need to monitor their health and be willing to seek professional help. They are responsible for ensuring their health problems do not affect patient care.

- Doctors must comply with occupational health and safety requirements, including recommended vaccination and testing requirements.

- Doctors who think they may have been exposed to a serious communicable disease must seek and follow advice from a suitably qualified colleague, such as a consultant in occupational health, infectious diseases, or public health, and, if found to be infected, have regular medical supervision.

- Doctors should avoid treating or prescribing for themselves, their family or close friends. They should be registered with a GP and consult their GP rather than deal with health problems alone or informally via colleagues.

DOCTORS TREATING THEIR OWN

As with all patients, sick health professionals want to be treated compassionately – with sensitivity, sympathy, empathy and non-judgmentally. However, trainers, employers and regulators often treat them as naughty schoolchildren or wrongdoers for crossing the boundary from practitioner to patient. Many in authority over doctors wrongly conflate illness with a performance issue, like a disciplinary issue that needs to be addressed. This is played out in over-disclosure, telling others *'In confidence, but just in case'*, until as with one patient at Practitioner Health, 17 different individuals (not including their secretaries) had been informed that a doctor was unwell and was a victim of domestic violence. Later, this doctor found that her details, including that she had been raped, were now on her training records to follow her through her career.

Doctors with jurisdiction over other doctors in training, mentoring, coaching or managerial positions do not need to do more than be empathetic and ensure that the unwell doctor is seeking appropriate help and as and when to support a return to work. Disclosure of personal information must be kept to a minimum and follow the Caldicott principles.

That doctors find it hard to treat doctors is not made any easier by the lack of guidance on what to expect and how to act. Where it does exist, for example, the GMC guidance, it is couched in the language of blame, harm and avoiding problems rather than concerning compassion, kindness and competence towards colleagues.

BOX 7.1: GMC advice

GENERAL MEDICAL COUNCIL GUIDANCE

You must protect patients from risk of harm posed by another colleague's conduct, performance or health. The safety of patients must come first at all times. If you have concerns that a colleague may not be fit to practice, you must take appropriate steps without delay, so that the concerns are investigated, and patients protected where necessary. This means you must give an honest explanation of your concerns to an appropriate person from your employing or contracting body and follow their procedures *Good Medical Practice* (2006), para 43.

If there are no appropriate local systems, or local systems do not resolve the problem, and you are still concerned about the safety of patients, you should inform the relevant regulatory body. If you are not sure what to do, discuss your concerns with an impartial colleague or contact your defence body, a professional organisation, or the GMC for advice (*Good Medical Practice* (2006), para 44). If you have management responsibilities, you should make sure that systems are in place through which colleagues can raise concerns about risks to patients, and you must follow the guidance in the GMC's 'Management for Doctors' (*Good Medical Practice* (2006), para 45).

Doctors themselves can inadvertently create barriers that deter their colleagues from seeking assistance. Treating fellow professionals often induces discomfort, a sentiment exacerbated by the hierarchical structure inherent in medicine, making consultation with more senior colleagues a particularly arduous task. The intricacies of discussing antidepressants' side effects and mechanisms with, say, a Professor of Psychopharmacology might evoke a sense of awkwardness. These doctors might harbour personal biases and presumptions about mental health and its treatment, which could significantly impede their ability to deliver appropriate care to their peers.

Moreover, preconceived notions about grappling with '*mental unwellness*' and its management can further compound the predicament. The wish to provide care to a fellow doctor can raise ethical dilemmas regarding the delicate balance of boundaries, confidentiality and potential conflicts of interest. Navigating these intricacies while ensuring effective treatment becomes imperative for doctors in such scenarios. However, they are not insurmountable, and if in doubt, treat any sick colleague as one would want to be treated oneself, with compassion and professionalism.

Furthermore, attending to a mentally distressed colleague can become tricky if both parties work or train in the same hospital training programme or share the same patients. This is almost inevitable when one considers how small the world of medicine is. This becomes even more pertinent in specialities such as mental health and general practice, where the treating health and the unwell health professionals are drawn from the same pool of clinicians. In such instances, maintaining objectivity and impartiality throughout the caregiving process is essential and flagging early in the caring/patient relationship that paths might cross in other roles.

So, the dynamics of doctors treating their fellow practitioners encapsulates multifaceted ethical and emotional challenges. For the treating doctor, regular supervision (such as attending a Balint group) can help to ensure competent and unbiased care.

The vignette below illustrates how best to treat a fellow health professional:

Rebecca, a psychiatrist, was referred by a colleague to care for a fellow doctor, Susan. Susan had been struggling with symptoms of depression and anxiety, impacting her personal life and professional performance. Recognising the unique dynamics of treating a fellow doctor, Rebecca approached the situation with empathy and understanding. During their initial session, Rebecca created a safe and non-judgmental environment for Susan to express her concerns and share her experiences. While apprehensive at first, Susan felt relieved to have someone who understood the challenges and pressures specific to the medical profession. As the consultations progressed, Susan began to disclose her feelings of burnout, imposter syndrome and the weight of responsibility that came with being a doctor. Rebecca carefully balanced her role as a treating doctor while being attuned to their shared professional background. Rebecca acknowledged the unique complexities of treating a fellow doctor, which included concerns about confidentiality, potential professional repercussions, and the need to establish boundaries. She reassured Susan that her confidentiality was paramount and that she would maintain strict professional limits to ensure privacy. Rebecca worked collaboratively with Susan throughout treatment to develop a treatment plan tailored to her needs. They explored various therapeutic modalities, such as cognitive-behavioural therapy and mindfulness techniques, to address her symptoms of depression and anxiety and to develop effective coping strategies for managing stress. During treatment, Rebecca remained mindful of the power dynamics and potential for transference and countertransference. She regularly checked in with Susan to ensure that their therapeutic relationship remained focused on Susan's needs and that any personal biases or experiences did not interfere with the treatment process.

Health professionals must resist taking shortcuts or jumping to assumptions when caring for other health professionals. The sick practitioner deserves the same explanations regarding the processes involved in investigating and managing their conditions. While their understanding of medical matters might surpass that of most patients, it is crucial not to presuppose the level of information and detail they need to deal with their health issues. This means explaining how and when to take medicines, expected side effects, what different psychological treatments entail, etc.

Encouraging doctors to engage in an ongoing doctor–patient relationship by attending routine follow-up appointments is essential. This way, they can maintain consistent care and address any changes or concerns that arise over time.

When treating doctors, being aware of one's emotional reactions and seeking clinical supervision or support as needed is essential. This can help mitigate the impact of countertransference and ensure that the therapeutic relationship remains focused on the patient's needs. Building trust and rapport with patients is essential, and this can be achieved through open communication, empathy and respect for the patient's autonomy.

BOX 7.2: Definitions of transference and countertransference

Transference involves the unconscious transfer of feelings, attitudes and desires from significant individuals in a person's past, typically from their early childhood, onto their therapist or another person in the present therapeutic relationship. Transference is considered a natural and common phenomenon in therapy and can significantly impact the therapeutic process.

Transference occurs when the patient unconsciously projects emotions and expectations onto the therapist associated with individuals from their past, such as parents, siblings, or authority figures. These projections can be positive or negative and may include feelings of love, anger, attachment, or romantic attraction. Transference can influence how the patient perceives and interacts with the therapist.

Therapists are trained to recognise and work with transference. They understand that the emotions and reactions expressed by the patient towards them often have roots in unresolved issues from the patient's past. By exploring and understanding these transference dynamics, therapists can help patients gain insight into their emotional and psychological patterns and work through unresolved conflicts. This process can be therapeutic and contribute to the patient's personal growth and self-awareness.

Countertransference refers to the health professionals' emotional reactions, attitudes and feelings towards a patient. It involves the health professionals' emotional response to them, which may be related to unresolved personal issues, biases, or past experiences. Countertransference can be positive or negative, impacting the therapeutic relationship and the treatment process.

Positive countertransference occurs when the health professional experiences positive emotions towards the patient, such as affection, admiration, or empathy. This can enhance the therapeutic relationship and contribute to the patient's progress. However, the clinician must maintain professional boundaries and ensure these positive feelings do not cloud their judgement or compromise the therapeutic process.

Negative countertransference involves the therapist experiencing negative emotions or reactions towards the patient. This could include feelings of frustration, anger, or irritation.

Negative countertransference may arise when the patient's issues trigger unresolved conflicts or issues in the therapist's life. Health professionals must recognise and manage negative countertransference to prevent it from adversely affecting the therapeutic encounter.

Those working in psychotherapy are trained to be aware of their countertransference reactions and to use them as valuable information to gain insights into their issues and potential blind spots. All clinicians are wise to think through potential countertransference with supervisors or colleagues to ensure that it doesn't interfere with the care they provide. Recognising and managing countertransference is important to maintaining professionalism and providing effective therapy.

Addressing psychological defences and building a solid therapeutic relationship is essential to effective treatment for doctors or other healthcare professionals with mental illness. By fostering an environment of trust and support, healthcare professionals can help their patients overcome their fears and work towards recovery.

This is best facilitated through clinical supervision and reflective practice. The modality of care might vary (for example, Balint Groups, reflective groups, work groups), but the overarching requirements are that it allows a space for the treating doctor, alone or in groups, to talk about their work in a safe, confidential and supportive space.

In reflective practice, healthcare professionals use self-awareness and self-evaluation to enhance their clinical practice. It involves critically analysing their thoughts, feelings, behaviours and patients' experiences to improve their professional knowledge and skills.

TIPS FOR TREATING DOCTORS WITH MENTAL ILLNESS

1. Be empathetic and understand the doctor's vulnerability and need for help and support.

2. Establish boundaries regarding what information can be disclosed and to whom.

3. Maintain professional boundaries and respect the time limits of appointments.

4. Avoid disclosing too much personal information about yourself to maintain the therapeutic relationship and avoid conflicts of interest.

5. Establish guidelines for handling situations where you may see the doctor outside the consulting room.

6. Be attentive to the doctor's symptoms and assess their condition carefully, as doctors may downplay them.

7. Avoid discussing medical politics or gossip and focus on the patient's needs.

8. Stick to your formulation and treatment plan while allowing the patient autonomy in the therapeutic process.

9. Encourage the doctor to register with a GP and facilitate necessary investigations or treatments.

10. Be mindful of potential countertransference reactions and professionally manage them.

PATIENTS, THE PUBLIC AND THEIR VIEWS OF SICK DOCTORS

Beyond the obvious of not wanting to wait longer for care, patients do not take kindly to unwell doctors. This is because it breaks their (the public's) belief that doctors are immune from illness. This is described in the literature. For example, the sociologist Talcott Parsons described the 'sick role' in terms of adopting certain expected behaviours and beliefs once unwell to maintain the boundary (consciously and unconsciously determined) between the doctor (*giver*) and patient (*taker*). He believed illness was a form of deviant behaviour within society because ill people cannot fulfil their expected social roles and thus move away from the consensual norm. Parsons devised the 'sick role mechanism' of how, ideally, a doctor and patient should interrelate. Within this mechanism, ill people and doctors had to abide by several 'rights' and 'obligations' attached to their respective roles. According to Parsons, the medical profession aims to return individuals to 'conventional' social roles. If this were not to happen, it would influence other institutions and could lead to a breakdown of the 'social body'.[64] Doctors are trained and expected not to become unwell. If they do, they are perceived as having deviated from socially prescribed normal behaviour, meaning that many either deny their illnesses in the first place or attend work when unwell. This is called 'presentism'.

The psychiatrist Thomas Main described the defensive interplay of projections between caregivers and patients and the 'phantastic' collusion.[65]

> *The helpful unconsciously requires others to be helpless, while the helpless will require others to be helpful. Staff and patients are thus inevitably, to some extent, creatures of each other.*

In this process, the nasty, frightening and distasteful aspect of illness can be projected into and contained (or held) within health professionals, who, given their training and status, accept these projections demanded of them by society. If a doctor becomes unwell, how can they hold this pain?

Both Parsons and Main describe that specific roles are ascribed to being a patient and a doctor, which have a basis in sociological and psychological theories. This creates an unconscious boundary which is extremely difficult to cross, which maintains the belief that *patients have the diseases, doctors wear magic white coats*.

Just as doctors form judgments about their patients, so patients form judgments about their doctors. These are based on cues such as appearance, demeanour, punctuality and communication style. These cues contribute to patients' interpretations of a doctor's well-being or illness.

Patients' perceptions of their doctors' health directly influence how they feel about the care they receive. When patients perceive their doctors as unwell, negative views can emerge, including perceptions of reduced competence, increased likelihood of errors and less appropriate interactions. Patients may also feel less comfortable and trusting of unwell doctors, potentially leading them to seek care from other healthcare providers.

8

Engagement, assessment and formulation

MAKING CONTACT

The initial contact with a health professional sets the foundation for building rapport, trust and honesty. However, as mentioned in this handbook, establishing an effective doctor–patient relationship can be challenging, as sick doctors may need help becoming dependent on the patient's role.

For many doctors, it might be their first-time seeking help for a mental health problem. They might feel ashamed, not just at being unwell but having to cross the divide between being the all-knowing doctor and the vulnerable patient. Removing their metaphorical white coat and putting on the patient gown can take some time. As a treating clinician, try not to rush these first stages.

Hassan arrived two hours and two minutes early for his first appointment. It wasn't unusual for doctors to be early for their first appointment; the combination of anxiety and their inbuilt perfectionism meant this was generally the norm. However, two hours and two minutes beat all records. Hassan had made himself known to the small office before this first appointment. He'd called the previous week asking for help, saying that it was urgent, 'You must help me', he screamed down the telephone, 'if you don't help me I will lose my job'.

His heavy accent and rapid speech made it difficult to understand him entirely, but the urgency of his distress came over. The first available appointment was given to him, and a confirmatory email was sent, 17.15 next Tuesday, four working days from now. He rang the following day to confirm the time, place and who he would see. He rang the day before the appointment to check if it was still happening, and he rang on the day to say that he was on his way but might be a little late as the traffic could have been better. He arrived for his appointment at 15:17; in his anxiety, he had misunderstood the 24-hour clock. His only option was to wait patiently.

DOI: 10.1201/9781003391500-8

Hassan might be exceptional in arriving so early for his appointment, but his anxiety reflects that of many others who seek help. This might be reflected in them attending before or maybe missing their initial appointment or wanting to use a pseudonym (though often using their email address with their full name).

Acknowledging the courage, difficulty and honesty of a doctor who accepts the patient's role is a crucial first step in engaging them in treatment. This helps create a supportive environment where the doctor feels understood and valued as a patient, promoting practical assessment and treatment.

THE CONSULTING ROOM

When doctors enter a consulting room, they tend to act differently, as they visibly try to regain control of their medical identity by, for example, *'talking shop'* or underplaying their symptoms. Sick doctors are often embarrassed when consulting with other doctors. A personal account called *'The other side of the sheets: a special case?'* was written by a doctor describing her experience of being admitted to a hospital with a physical problem.[66] She writes:

> I recount my experience, not going for sympathy, but to make the point that doctors are 'special patients'. From the start, I presented late with a list of differential diagnoses rather than symptoms. Fear of a laparotomy made the abdominal pain 'not too bad' or 'tolerable' rather than 'awful.' Conscious of the overworked nurses, I ignored that I'd had morphine and was found in a heap on the floor, and the night passed in morose tears and indescribable morbid fears. Also, as a doctor, I could not ignore my fellow patients.

This anonymous account illustrates how sick doctors can differ from other patients. They often present late and then with diagnoses rather than saying what is wrong with them, *'This is wrong with me'*, rather than *'I have a pain in my foot'*. They minimise their symptoms, such as deliberately scoring lower on alcohol screening questionnaires or masking the true extent of their negative thinking. This handbook has already discussed some issues interfering with the doctor–patient relationship where the patient is a doctor. The treating doctor might worry about the manner of treating a colleague and perhaps have concerns about navigating complex regulatory issues. Real challenges might be involved, such as understanding confidentiality or reporting requirements. There could even be legal repercussions if the sick doctor makes an error at work whilst under their care. Then, there is the scenario where the treating doctor might have a professional relationship with the doctor they are caring for, further creating problems of maintaining appropriate boundaries and objectivity. Addressing these concerns with the patient and reassuring them that there are confidentiality and sharing agreements can help alleviate some of these worries and create a safe environment for doctors seeking treatment.

This can be done in the first instance by:

- Building a working relationship
- Showing that you care
- Working towards mutually acceptable goals
- Building rapport
- Building trust

These can often be achieved/aided by:

- Explaining and providing confidentiality
- Interviewing individually
- An appropriate setting
- A flexible approach
- Being non-confrontational
- Being non-judgmental
- Not assuming the worst: It is rare for a sick doctor to harm a patient

UNDERSTANDING DUAL RESPONSIBILITIES

Looking after a sick doctor involves assuming dual responsibility. In the first instance, and as with other non-medical patients, the treating clinician has a duty of care towards their patient. Secondly, not as obviously, the treating doctor is also carrying out an occupational risk assessment due to the safety-conscious nature of medicine. The patient's care is still the doctor's primary concern, and one must be mindful of the responsibilities of attending to a patient who is also a health professional. This will be discussed in more detail later in this handbook regarding the need to share information.

SETTING AND MAINTAINING BOUNDARIES

Boundaries are essential in all clinical encounters, and doctors across all disciplines must understand how and what to do to maintain them. Typically, this would include setting time boundaries, seeing patients only in designated health sites, restricting sharing personal information, and (trying) not meeting patients in social or professional situations. All of these become difficult when the patient is a doctor and when doctors consult with each other. As said earlier, the world of medicine is small, and connections between treating and sick doctors often happen. These must be managed, and it is best to acknowledge these links rather than ignore them. Treating doctors must ensure that they maintain patient confidentiality and not disclose sensitive information to others unless directly involved in their care or where there are overriding reasons to do so. This would mean not discussing their patient in case conferences, learning events, articles, or books without full consent. It is striking how often doctors breach confidentiality, discussing 'an interesting case' in canteens, conferences and with friends over dinner. No wonder sick doctors are anxious about attending for care.

Maintaining boundaries is essential to ensure professionalism and provide containment. It goes beyond confidentiality and statutory obligations and involves establishing clear parameters for the consultation. This includes setting appointment times and limits, agreed contact methods, perhaps even the use of titles, and limited self-disclosure.

In the case of treating other doctors, the need for boundary vigilance becomes even more crucial due to the potential for social or professional overlap. When doctors treat their colleagues, they are more likely to encounter them outside the therapeutic context. Upholding a professional relationship from the beginning helps to mitigate anxieties that may arise in such situations. It is helpful to rehearse how any interaction might be played out if the treating and the treated doctors meet in a work or social environment (which, given the nature of medicine, is not uncommon). In any event, it is not for the treating doctor to disclose their therapeutic relationship. It is surprising how many practitioner–patients choose to talk publicly about their mental illness, sometimes even verging on over-disclosure. Talking about the limits of maintaining personal boundaries and ones between their clinicians might help avoid over-disclosure.

INITIAL ASSESSMENT

Regardless of whether the patient is a health professional, the assessment process follows a similar path. During the consultation, the clinician aims to elicit information about the patient's presenting complaint, precipitating factors (why now?), predisposing factors (factors that make the patient susceptible to developing the problem), perpetuating factors (factors that might impede recovery) and protective factors (factors that might enhance recovery now and, in the future).

During the first contact, the health professional tries to understand and formulate the presenting issues in the context of their personal and professional life into an understandable narrative. As time and contact goes on, this formulation can be added to.

Some questions to consider asking may include the following:

1. Why did the individual choose to pursue medicine as a career? This question can help to understand personal and family history, including whether other doctors were in the family and whether the choice was freely made or due to parental pressure.

2. How was medical school and further training? This can help to tease out any problems to date, including issues with studying, passing exams, interpersonal relationships and whether the individual has created a professional support network and professional identity.

3. Have there been any breaks in training or service, and if so, why did these occur?

4. What is the current work situation, including any work in the NHS, private practice, or academic medicine?

5. What is the person's medical and psychiatric history, including addictive behaviours?

6. Has the individual been involved with complaints, significant events or referrals to regulators?

7. Are there any financial problems, including reasons why? Doctors tend to be well-paid, but they may also spend beyond their means and borrow money based on future earnings. This can lead to significant financial stress and impact mental health.

It is also good to ask open-ended questions to allow the patient to provide as much detail as possible while still being mindful of time constraints. Additionally, assess the patient's mental state and risk of harm to themselves or others. Finally, provide the patient with information about their diagnosis, treatment options and any potential side effects or risks associated with treatment.

Irrespective of what practitioner–patients presented for care, all patients should be asked the following:

- Any gaps in work/education
- Substance use history
- Whether any current complaints
- Whether in debt
- Suicidal thoughts
- Contact number for 'In Case of Emergency' (ICE)

FORMULATION

In the context of patient assessment, developing a formulation refers to a comprehensive understanding of a patient's medical, psychological and social factors contributing to their health condition or concerns. This formulation helps make informed diagnosis, treatment and care planning decisions. It is essential in psychiatry, psychology and complex medical cases.

By integrating these factors into a coherent patient formulation, healthcare providers can develop a more holistic and individualised understanding of the patient's condition. This, in turn, enables them to create a tailored treatment plan that addresses the patient's unique needs and circumstances. It's a collaborative process aiming to provide the most effective patient-centred care. This is summarised in Figure 8.1.

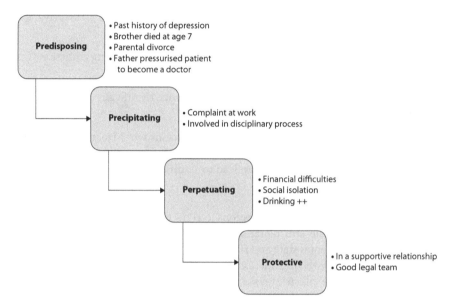

Figure 8.1 Formulation.

9

Suicide risk and management

Suicidal thoughts usually start when someone feels overwhelmed by problems or their situation. If a practitioner–patient is considering suicide, they do not necessarily want their life to end; instead, when asked, they want to escape from intolerable distress and see suicide as the only option open to them at the time.

Several psychological processes may make a person more prone to self-harm and suicide. Losses and abandonment in relationships are common precipitants in both self-harm and suicide. Additionally, defeat, humiliation and entrapment, when the person sees no positive future and way out of their current situation, are predictors of suicidal behaviour.

ASSESSING RISK

Most people who die by suicide have a mental disorder, although the presence of suicidal thoughts is not always a feature of mental illness, and having a mental illness rarely leads to suicide. Suicide is rare, yet suicidal thoughts and mental illness are prevalent. Hence, it is extremely difficult to determine who might end their life, even if they have the most severe mental illness or pervasive thoughts of death. Suicidal thoughts and feelings can occur in anyone, whether they have a mental illness or not, and develop in response to emotional distress or despair. Mental illness is more strongly associated with suicidal ideation than with suicide attempts. Research indicates that psychiatric risk factors are poor predictors of suicidal behaviour.[67]

Other than genuine sadness at the loss of life, what worries treating doctors, perhaps more than anything else when treating a patient with mental illness, is that their patient might take their own life and that they will be held responsible for the death. The assessing or treating clinician is often blamed (and accepts this blame) without understanding that predicting who might or might not kill themselves is challenging. Despite what might be said later in coroners' courts, reliable prediction is rarely possible. It is worth repeating suicide is a rare event, and the

DOI: 10.1201/9781003391500-9

potential risk factors are prevalent; therefore, identifying the person who will go on to kill themselves amongst those who express suicidal thoughts or feelings of hopelessness is very difficult.

Suicidal intent can also change rapidly, hence the scenario of seeing the patient in the morning, doing a careful assessment, with the individual then going on to take their own life later in the day. This is not to say that a risk assessment should not be undertaken; rather, one should be mindful that this risk assessment is not conflated with suicide prediction.

Assessing doctors can be complicated as they will be alert to questions to elucidate risk and might even cover up by giving falsely reassuring answers. It is not uncommon for doctors to minimise their symptoms, consciously or unconsciously, to deny the extent of their depressed mood or even the presence of hallucinations or delusion beliefs. There is also the ongoing problem of resistance to accepting the patient role, which is associated with shame, failure and guilt. It is sadly well known for a doctor to present a 'positive front' to the assessing clinician, only to take their own life soon after.

Suicide is a complex and multifaceted issue, and there is rarely a single cause or explanation. Intent to kill oneself lies on a continuum from the more common vague, passive suicidal thoughts to the rarer, suicidal acts. To try and assess where someone is on this continuum is hard.

In clinical practice, concern about suicide risk begins with one or more of the following situations:

- Recognition that a patient is seriously distressed or mentally unwell

- A clear or covert statement indicating that the patient is considering suicide; for example, *'I'm not sure how long I can go on like this'* or *'I'm just so tired of being down'*

- Communication from a family member or friend concerned about the patient; for example, *'He keeps talking about how we'd be better off without him'*

Asking some simple questions (as below) can open a dialogue.

- *'Have things got so bad that you've thought about hurting yourself or ending your life?'*

- *Tell me about your suicidal thoughts.*

Remember that asking about suicidal intent does not plant the idea in the patient's head. Instead, asking why now and identifying the final straw can help target interventions to reduce risk. A calm, non-judgmental, concerned approach tells the patient that you care and will be able to cope with the answers.

If the patient says they are having suicidal thoughts, then the next step is to try and find out how serious the suicidal intent is by asking:

- *'What kinds of thoughts have you been having?'*
- *'How long have you been having these thoughts? When did they first start?'*
- *'How often are these thoughts happening? Daily? Weekly? All the time?'*

And then whether they have made a definitive plan and have access to the means:

- *'Do you have a plan for how you would kill yourself?'*
- *'Have you thought about any other methods?'*
- *'Do you have any tablets at home?'*
- *'Have you "rehearsed" or "gone through the motions" of killing yourself?'*

Screening tests are usually brief and easy to use, and they can help begin a problematic discussion or focus further questioning. Still, they must be kept from being relied on as they have a high rate of false positives and a low positive predictive value compared with the gold standard of the psychiatric interview.

EIGHT TRUTHS ABOUT SUICIDE

The psychiatrist and one of the leading experts on suicide, Rachel Gibbons, has elucidated her views on suicide and helpfully created 'eight rules' about the subject.[68]

These 'truths' came about following her own experience when two patients killed themselves unwell in her care when she had just started her consultant post and after hearing stories of deaths by suicide and of clinicians' emotional responses to them.

The following 'truths' are adapted from her paper:

1. Suicide is not an accident. Instead, it is due to a complex interplay of factors, including genetic predisposition, exposure and outcome of early trauma and recent life events.

2. One will never know why someone died by suicide as the person who could have shed some light on the situation is no longer present. Even when people have been interviewed after making a serious attempt on their lives, they are frequently unclear as to why they did it and can be as shocked as everyone else by their actions.

3. Suicide is an 'acting out' behaviour that results in death. 'Acting out' is an unconscious defence mechanism where action takes the place of feeling. For

many who make severe attempts on their life, the first sign that they feel in such overwhelming distress is that they act.

4. Everyone is shocked by the death of an individual through suicide. The National Confidential Inquiry found that each year, around 73% of people who die by suicide have not been in touch with mental health services in the year preceding their death. For 27% who had had a risk assessment tool filled in at their last contact, 83% have been rated as no or low risk. Even in the small group with recognised severe ongoing suicidality, there is often no expectation of the attempt. Some patients are even reported to appear to improve before their death.

5. Suicide appears to be either impulsive or premeditated. In other words, some individuals meticulously plan their deaths, even to the extent of having a *dress rehearsal* beforehand. For others, it appears to be completely impulsive, occurring, for example, following an argument.

6. Suicide is part of the human condition and is not just related to mental health problems. The relationship between suicide and mental illness is complicated and poorly understood. Many people do not have a diagnosed mental illness at the time of death, and some have no history of mental distress.

7. One cannot read other people's minds. We do not know what happens in our mind often, as around 90% of its functioning is unconscious. In mental health services, however, there is an underlying omnipotent belief, supported by societal expectations, that mental health professionals (and one could attest, also general practitioners and those assessing patients in accident and emergency departments) have a special intuition about others' minds and can predict an action someone else is going to make in the future.

8. No one is to blame for someone else's death by suicide. This is perhaps the most important truth. No matter how much the treating clinician blames themselves for their patient's death, it is not their fault, and to think so is magical thinking.

SUICIDE RISK FACTORS IN DOCTORS

Rachel Gibbons argues in her article[48] that:

> Concern about suicide cannot just be focused on those working in mental health, giving them the impossible task of predicting the unpredictable and controlling the uncontrollable. The focus on risk assessment and prediction of suicide in mental health settings sets a goal that we can only fail in. It also distracts us from our primary task of therapeutic engagement to improve quality of life.

This does not negate the need to try and identify and modify risk factors, but their presence does not solely determine suicidal behaviour. What is as important is an individual's ability to cope with stress and adversity and the availability of protective factors to mitigate the risk of suicide.

Clinicians must not rely wholly on identifying risk factors when assessing individuals. A person may be at an elevated or increased chance of suicide even though they are not known to be in an at-risk group and, conversely, not all members of high-risk groups are at equal risk of suicide. The most substantial risk factors for acting on suicidal thoughts in high-income countries are previous suicidal behaviour and a mood disorder, particularly if accompanied by substance abuse, gambling addiction and stressful life events. The presence of 'red flag' warning signs suggests that someone may be particularly at risk of suicide. However, risk factors and red flag warning signs should not be used to predict or rule out an individual suicide (or attempt).

Whilst doctors share risk factors for suicide with their non-doctor patients (such as traumatic life events, gambling, drug or alcohol abuse), they also have additional issues which place them at risk.

These include the following.

Life events

It is impossible to avoid life events such as moving to a new house, divorce, illness and so on, contributing to the pathogenesis of mental illness. Doctors must move frequently due to training rotations and career progression. Moving disrupts social networks and increases the risk of doctors feeling isolated and unable to know where to seek help and support.

Isolation and loneliness

Loneliness has been likened to experiencing hunger, which signals a person to seek out food. Likewise, feeling momentarily lonely may prompt a person to seek out connections, which, in evolutionary terms, would be advantageous. In this sense, many people will report having experienced brief periods of loneliness from time to time. However, *persistent* loneliness is associated with several poor health outcomes, including mental health. Doctors who work unsocial hours and night shifts, moving frequently and under stress, may find this interferes with their ability to maintain relationships, make new connections or keep in touch with family. They also, especially if working as locums, live in on-call or hospital residences, with little or no contact with others, all passing like ships in the night. Loneliness is associated with depression, psychosis, cognitive impairment, dementia, suicidal ideation and completed suicide. Medicine can be a lonely business. Isolation creeps in through every door. There is professional isolation from peers, colleagues and seniors at work. There is social isolation from loved ones and friends at home. There is mental or physical isolation from illness and disability. Doctors can find themselves surrounded by people and yet very much alone.

Access to drugs

Analysis of suicide risk by specialities is somewhat limited due to relatively small numbers of deaths in different categories. However, many studies find a higher risk for anaesthetists and a lower risk for paediatricians. This is predicated on anaesthetists and other doctors working in critical care or emergency departments with easy access to potent drugs.

Self-harm versus suicidality

Although most people who self-harm do not intend to end their lives, self-harm increases the likelihood of future suicide, so every episode of self-harm must be taken seriously.

Not all patients who harm themselves are actively suicidal. To differentiate self-harm from suicidal behaviour, one must ask about the patient's intentions. Was the behaviour (e.g., cutting, burning) done to end their life, relieve emotional distress or overcome a feeling of numbness? Remember, though, that self-harm patients may have more than one intention for the behaviour, and self-harm is a risk factor for future suicide attempts. The co-existence of both behaviours is common in personality disorder.

Some clinicians may see suicide prevention as outside their remit, but suicide **can be prevented** until the end. The key is compassion, safeguarding, safety planning, hope and mitigating risk factors whilst addressing mental illness and life crises.

MANAGING THE SUICIDAL PATIENT

Christine, a junior doctor, struggled with coming to work on time. She found shift work coupled with long-standing insomnia challenging to cope with. Her occupational health nurse has advised Christine to seek help from Practitioner Health. She has a long history of low mood and anxiety and is taking antidepressants. You manage to elicit that she is sad but can't/won't give you any more details. She denies suicidal ideation by shaking her head but sighs or shrugs her shoulders when you ask her questions to find out more. She does not take drugs (she says anyway) but smelled very strongly of alcohol during the assessment. She lives in a house share but reports that she does not know her flatmates and keeps herself to herself. She is currently working and reports that no concerns have been raised about her ability/health. When asked why she was seen at occupational health, she shrugs and says she does not know. You are very concerned about her risk to herself and her patients in her current state. She doesn't want to go on sick leave as she feels work gives her a purpose and means she must get up in the morning.

As a treating doctor, it is hard not to have serious concerns about Christine's mental health and her risk of self-harm. She is isolated, has numbed herself with alcohol and seems disinterested in herself and her predicament. Her only protective factor is her work – even here, you have concerns about her fitness to practise. Asking her to take leave might be the tipping point of suicidal behaviour. It is unlikely that Christine meets any criteria for compulsory admission and would more than likely refuse voluntary admission into the hospital. She does need safety netting, including determining who she might be able to call/visit if feeling so low that she might consider taking her own life, what emergency services she might be able to access, including out-of-hours GP services, accident and emergency and the Samaritans. Depending on the service arrangements, engaging a home treatment or crisis team might be appropriate. Getting consent to contact others who might be able to support her would also help, as would arranging to make contact soon after this consultation.

Chandra lived in hospital accommodation. He had recently started work as a maternity locum in accident and emergency. His family live in Kuwait, and he came to work in England a few years ago. It is hard now for him to return. Chandra had recently been suspended after a complaint from a patient who said he had been rude to her and shouted. He denies this, saying he had been upset as the patient had been racist and said she didn't want to see a foreign doctor. Even before this, he had noticed how irritable he had become and had lost interest in most things. All he seemed to do was work. He had no friends, family in England or social network. He started to cry. He said he would be better off dead.

Chandra is at increased risk for suicide, with many areas of concern. He lives alone in hospital accommodation. He is socially isolated and depressed and has a significant risk factor in the complaint and subsequent suspension from work. Having identified him as being high risk, it is essential to determine the level of risk and to ensure what plans are made for his safety, including the possible need for admission.

In the main, suicide risk can be reduced through good communication, empathy, appropriate treatment (such as antidepressants or behavioural treatment), access to support and therapy groups, and recruiting significant others to help support the doctor during this time. For some doctors, it might be necessary to escalate one's concerns and involve other health professionals or, rarely, even consider admission (voluntary or under the Mental Health Act).

Even if the health professional does not disclose suicidal thoughts or has not yet developed them, it is essential to consider co-producing a safety plan should they become suicidal. Making such a safety plan builds a patient's resilience and resourcefulness to confront any potential suicidal thoughts resulting from new life events, recurrences of distress or a worsening of a mental illness.

RESOURCES

1. Connecting with People.[48]

2. Stay Alive suicide prevention app for smartphones and tablets can be downloaded from the Apple App Store or Google Play.

3. *You are feeling on edge helping you get through it* – for people in distress attending the emergency department following self-harm or with suicidal thoughts:

   - *www.rcpsych.ac.uk/healthadvice/problemsdisorders/feelingontheedge.aspx*

10

Impact of complaints

COMPLAINTS

Mental illness and suicide are risks for doctors undergoing any disciplinary investigation. This is a long-standing concern. For example, in 1976, the Oregon Board of Medical Examiners (equivalent to the UK General Medical Council) became uneasy about the high rate of suicide among doctors who were under regulatory supervision. In 13 months, 8 out of 40 doctors involved with their processes had killed themselves. All the doctors had a history of severe, undiagnosed mental illness, namely depression and tended to be socially isolated.[69] Decades later, this time in the UK, concerns were raised about the high rates of suicide among doctors passing through regulatory processes. The General Medical Council (GMC) commissioned an independent study to examine the 28 deaths due to suicide (or suspected suicide) among doctors involved in fitness-to-practise processes between 2005 and 2013. The case reviews of these doctors showed that many suffered from a recognised mental health disorder, including drug and alcohol addictions. Other factors, which often follow from those conditions, may have also contributed to their deaths. These included marriage breakdown, financial hardship and, in some cases, police involvement, as well as the stress of being involved in a disciplinary process.[7,70]

Although correlation does not equal causation, being under regulatory or disciplinary processes or having a complaint nevertheless increases the risk of mental illness among doctors. This is due to the complaint or referral itself and its protracted nature. Severe criticism can take years to pass through the various processes, and multiple jeopardies are common. Numerous investigations, including employer disciplinary processes, can take many years, exacerbating any pre-existing mental health problem and being a significant precipitant for new-onset mental illness.

Researchers have found that doctors who had recently received a complaint were 77% more likely to suffer from moderate to severe depression than those who had never had a complaint. They were also found to have more suicidal thoughts, sleep difficulties, relationship problems and a host of physical health problems compared to doctors who had not been through a complaints process. Those without a complaint had suicidal thoughts at around 2.5%, which increased to about 9% for those with a current or recent complaint and 13% for those with a past complaint. Poorly handled complaints often result in dysfunctional behaviours, such as failure to disclose all events, blaming of self and others and arguments, which can contribute to doctors killing themselves. Even minor complaints can significantly impact doctors and be a powerful trigger for mental illness and suicide.[71,72]

Phillipa was only 26 when she ended her life a few weeks after she had received a complaint. She was left demoralised and ashamed that she had failed as a doctor. She feared she would lose her job. Instead, she lost her life. The poor handling of her complaint, the delays, the assumption of blame and the lack of support (practical and emotional) were significant contributors to her suicide. And she is not alone.

Complaints against doctors are shared and on the rise. Most complaints relate to clinical issues and poor communication, which increases when a doctor is tired, or work intensity makes it hard to focus.

The reasons why complaints are so difficult are varied and include the following:

1. **Professional identity and self-worth:** Many doctors have a robust professional identity and derive a sense of self-worth from their work. When they receive a complaint, it can challenge their perception of themselves as competent and caring professionals. It may lead to self-doubt, inadequacy and a blow to their professional identity.

2. **Emotional impact:** Doctors often form emotional connections with their patients, particularly in long-term care or critical situations. When a patient complains, it can be emotionally distressing for the doctor if they have invested significant time and effort into providing the best care possible. The sense of betrayal or loss of trust can be deeply hurtful.

3. **Fear of legal and professional consequences:** Complaints can trigger anxiety and fear of legal or professional repercussions. Doctors may worry about being sued, damaging their professional reputations, disciplinary actions by regulators or employers, or potentially impacting their careers. The uncertainty surrounding the outcome of a complaint can contribute to stress and psychological distress.

4. **Stigma and isolation:** The experience of being complained about may carry a stigma within the medical community. Doctors may fear judgement and ostracisation from colleagues, which can intensify feelings of shame and isolation. The perceived loss of support and trust within their professional network can exacerbate mental health challenges.

5. **Cumulative effect:** If doctors face multiple complaints or a history of complaints, it can negatively impact their mental health. Repeated exposure to negative feedback or complaints can contribute to chronic stress, burnout and feeling overwhelmed. Over time, this can erode their job satisfaction and contribute to mental health problems.

RELATIONSHIP BETWEEN MENTAL ILLNESS IN DOCTORS AND COMPLAINTS

- A complaint may make a doctor depressed or worsen a pre-existing mental condition.

- Mental illness can lead to cognitive impairment, boundary transgression or inappropriate behaviour, such as bullying or acting inappropriately with a patient or work colleague.

- Mental illness might lead to out-of-character criminal behaviour (such as shoplifting), worsening mental illness.

- Mental illness might be a criminal activity, the most apparent drug use.

- Drug use can lead doctors to transgress good medical practice, such as stealing drugs or self-prescribing or prescribing in a patient's name for the doctor's use.

- Mental illness might be considered counter to fitness to practise, for example, bipolar disorder, schizophrenia, personality disorder or schizoaffective disorder.

- Trying to kill oneself might lead to criminal or professional sanctions where the means of the suicide attempt involves obtaining drugs illegally or via self-prescription.

DEALING WITH COMPLAINTS

A doctor from Practitioner Health's patient group has written this guidance about what to do if you receive a complaint.

- Stop, think and take a deep breath. This is not about you or your personality. This is about the system and the patient. You are not a bad person because you have received a complaint.

- Do not send any emails in haste – to anyone.

- If it is a serious complaint, ring your medical defence organisation; this will give you the earliest opportunity to get a legal view of the complaint and how to proceed. Ask your medical director, supervisor, trainer or colleague. In other words, seek advice.

- If you are a general practitioner (GP), depending on the nature of the complaint, you should also contact your local medical committee for further support and advice.

- Talk to your friends/peers. Put the complaint in perspective. Your peers can provide support moving forward and give you a balanced view of the complaint itself.

- Use your support networks you have, whether that be family or friends – just talking it through with someone can give a different perspective.

- Keep a contemporaneous diary of events – this will be useful to you as the complaint progresses.

- Be prepared for a long process; complaints can often take several months or even years to be investigated, so comply fully with them – let them know of any annual leave and respond promptly to their correspondence.

- Look after yourself – these investigations can be demanding physically, emotionally and psychologically – visit your GP and get the help you need.

- Remember, you are not the only one going through this. The regulator receives over 10,000 complaints each year against UK doctors, so do not isolate yourself; use the support that you have available.

11

Mental illness and professionalism

This chapter examines the regulatory process and its relevance to health-related cases. However, it is crucial not to rely solely on what is written, as guidelines evolve with time, and regulatory requirements may change. When a doctor is involved in any disciplinary procedure or investigation, seeking legal assistance is imperative. Doctors responsible for the care of these colleagues should possess some awareness, especially regarding potential challenges their patients might encounter.

The role of the treating doctor is to help alleviate some of their patient's anxiety, ensuring that the patient follows the guidance of their legal representative and that they remain a source of support throughout what might be an extended legal process.

When treating mentally ill doctors, one needs to be mindful of the interface between the doctor, their illness and their (that is, the sick doctors) duties as a clinician. Most health practitioners are in a safety-critical role; what they do can have a major impact on others, even if they do not work in a patient-facing role.

RECEIVING A COMPLAINT

When a doctor receives a notice indicating they are under investigation or facing a potentially serious complaint, their initial reaction is sheer panic. And in this state of high anxiety, they might not act in their best interests. For example, they might attend interviews unaccompanied and unprepared and not, as they should, engage legal advice ahead of any formal (or even informal) meeting. It is not unknown for doctors to 'over disclose', such that they admit to things which they have not done (such as failing to check on a patient) or to rely on their memory for the management of their patient instead of asking for the case notes to look at. The more serious the complaint, the more important it is to take time, ask for advice, remain silent and not feel coerced into attending an interview with senior staff members.

Joseph, a GP working in an Urgent Care Center, had just finished a 14-hour night shift at work and received a text from his duty manager that there had been a complaint from one of the patients he had attended that night. He was asked to return to work that morning to meet with the medical director (MD). After a quick shower and breakfast, he returned to work and, in the car, tried hard to go through all the patients he had seen that night. It had been busy, but not more so than usual. He met the MD as instructed and was surprised that the head of human resources was also present. He began to panic. What had he done? The MD began to explain that a female patient had complained that he had been sexually inappropriate and that he had placed his hand on her breast during a chest examination. The complainant also said that he had commented about the size of her breasts. Joseph remembered the consultation. A young woman with asthma, nothing much, but he listened to her chest, front and back, and had asked her if she wanted a chaperone, which she had refused. He had not touched her breasts, not that he remembered anyway, and certainly would not have made a comment. But what should he do now?

In a panic, he blurted out

'sorry....I can't remember. ...but if I did.... it's not what I normally do....and I didn't mean anything......sorry'.

Joseph was suspended from work, and that he had made this admission was later used in evidence against him at a subsequent tribunal. He should have asked ahead of time what it was about. If he did attend unprepared (as he had), he could have listened and then, before making any comments, asked to reconvene once he had obtained advice and legal representation as appropriate. He should also not have been asked to attend after he had rested and not after a long night shift and requested the meeting be delayed until he could be refreshed.

Whilst this is a fictional case, it is based on many doctors who have attended PH. Doctors are trained and expected to be honest and open in all their dealings. But they are also citizens with rights, including being seen as innocent before being proven guilty and having access to support and professional representation when serious issues arise.

BOX 11.1: What to do in the case of a serious complaint

PROMPTLY SEEK GUIDANCE

Seek advice at the earliest opportunity.

Contact your medical defence organisation (MDO) immediately. They are available 24/7.

Furthermore, remember:

- The initial call may necessitate subsequent written communication, such as a report detailing the events, copies of relevant medical records and updates on developments.

- Serious patient safety incidents, particularly those resulting in a patient's death, can lead to various medico-legal challenges.
- Having access to expert advice right from the start is imperative.

MAINTAINING CLINICAL RECORDS

Despite the distress and anxiety associated with a severe patient safety incident, it is essential to maintain accurate and contemporaneous records of the events and actions in the medical records.

Never alter a clinical record without a very good reason. For example, if you need to add something in the record which you had forgotten initially, then make sure it is clear that you have done this retrospectively and listed the reasons 'why'. Doctors can get into serious trouble for amending records to try and avert attention from something had or had not done.

On rare occasions where additions are necessary, they must be made formally as post-dated entries, but it is advisable to consult your MDO before doing so.

DRAFTING A DETAILED ACCOUNT

The account post-event might differ from the clinical record. This is not unusual as clinical records are not written in the event of 'just in case something bad happens'.

Write an account of what you think has happened as soon as possible, ideally within the first 24 hours, whilst still fresh in your mind. This is a painful process as one's natural inclination is to hide away and not to think about the serious event.

Compose a chronological account of what transpired, including conversations with others, advice received and discussions had with patients or relatives.

The report is a factual narrative, not one's personal opinions and conjectures, and will serve as the basis for subsequent medico-legal reports and statements.

DUTY OF CANDOUR

Our professional duty of candour applies whenever an error occurs, causing harm or distress to a patient.

Patients and their families expect an explanation of what went wrong (or as much as is known), an apology and a plan for corrective actions. Being transparent with patients is ethically sound and the right thing to do. Speak to your MDO for advice if you are worried about the implications of a duty of candour disclosure.

SEEK SUPPORT FOR MEETINGS

Your medical director or another senior manager will likely want to meet to discuss the next steps. In this case, seeking advice from your medical defence organisation or the British Medical Association before the meeting is important. Consider bringing an advocate or a senior colleague to any meeting.

SECOND VICTIM

The Royal College of Surgeons has published a guide to good practice in supporting surgeons after an adverse event. The document introduces the concept of the '**second victim**' after a serious adverse event. This term has attracted controversy as it might diminish the impact on the first victim (that is, the patient or their carer). However, whatever descriptor is used, the concept is simple: Healthcare providers involved in an adverse event commonly suffer psychologically and professionally. Their social interactions may be negatively impacted, and mental or physical health problems may develop or be exacerbated.

The work done in producing their report found that surgeons dealing with the aftermath of an adverse event may find themselves at a heightened risk of making subsequent errors. In the UK, data reveals that adverse events profoundly impact surgeons, leading to feelings of guilt, excessive worry, rumination and crises of confidence. Moreover, a national survey between 2016 and 2019 unveiled a high prevalence of post-traumatic stress symptoms among UK surgeons, akin to the rates experienced by military personnel returning from conflict zones. This survey, coupled with numerous anecdotal reports, underscores the pressing need for guidance to help surgeons and their employers navigate the multifaceted issues arising from an adverse event.

Specifically, surgeons have articulated several key concerns:

- Knowledge of the appropriate steps following an adverse event is needed.
- There needs to be a clear timeline for resolution.
- Limited emotional and practical support for affected surgeons.
- Scarce guidance for those desiring to offer support.
- Overemphasis on statutory responsibilities, investigations or disciplinary procedures, with insufficient attention to the well-being of the surgeon involved.
- Uncertainty surrounding the surgeon's continued practice and the necessary support for their return to work.

Following an adverse event, many stakeholders can become involved: The doctors themselves, their clinical or medical director, the employing organisation, their medical defence organisation, their trade union, the college or speciality association. Each of these stakeholders may have specific responsibilities and insights to contribute. Simultaneously, the doctor faces numerous personal and professional challenges, such as attending to the immediate needs of the patient or their caregivers, dealing with the emotional impact, concerns about their professional reputation, confidence issues, fears and uncertainty regarding complaints and litigation, and questions regarding when and how to resume work and under what circumstances.

- RCS England - Supporting surgeons after adverse events: *https://www.rcseng. ac.uk/standards-and-research/standards-and-guidance/good-practice-guides/ supporting-surgeons-after-adverse-events/guide/*

PROFESSIONAL BEHAVIOUR

Knowing what constitutes professional behaviour is one thing, but consistently demonstrating professionalism amid the pressures of a busy medical practice with conflicting demands and multiple goals is another. Professionalism is a learned skill that improves over time, and it is more about a spectrum of behaviours than an all-or-nothing trait. Distinguishing between doctors' professional and unprofessional behaviour hinges on their habits, as even the most skilled practitioners can have behavioural lapses.

Medical professionalism embodies altruism, accountability, commitment to excellence, duty, service, honour and respect for others. It serves as the cornerstone of the doctor–society relationship. Professionalism aspires to excellence, setting high standards and objectives, which is a reasonable expectation. However, an excessive pursuit of perfection can result in fatigue, stress, despair and a decline in academic or work performance. Consequently, professionals grappling with poor mental well-being find it challenging to engage fully in their work, often adopting a pessimistic and cynical outlook towards their patients and their profession.[70] Diminished mental well-being, characterised by fatigue, stress, depression, anxiety and overall reduced quality of life, has been linked to decreased medical professionalism, particularly in terms of empathy.[20]

However, whilst mental illness is linked to diminished empathy, there is little evidence that mental illness leads to actual harm to patients (though one could argue that lack of an empathic clinical encounter is harmful). This is not to say that a doctor with *active* or *unadressed* addiction is good for patient care; far from it. However, there is no robust evidence in the literature that equates mental illness leads to poor patient care.

Impaired physician

Concerns around mental illness and fitness to practise (FTP) often revolve around substance misuse, and it was addressing substance misuse in doctors that the Physician Health Programmes were started in the USA. They introduced the term '*impaired physician*', which characterises medical professionals facing health (mental or physical) problems that affect their ability to practise effectively. The American Medical Association initially defined an impaired physician in the 1970s as someone incapable of meeting their professional or personal obligations due to psychiatric disorders, alcoholism or drug dependence. This definition has since been broadened.

> An impaired physician is defined as *'any physical, mental, or behavioural condition that hinders the safe engagement in professional activities'.*

This updated perspective acknowledges that various conditions can hinder the execution of medical duties, irrespective of the doctor's knowledge and skills.

Mental health problems might affect a doctor's judgement, decision-making abilities, interpersonal skills or overall functioning, potentially leading to transgressions of professional conduct.

Examples of the interface between mental illness and professional practice

Whilst not exaggerating the risk that mental illness can have on their own patient's care, there is, however, an overlap between professionalism or violations of General Medical Practice Good Medical Practice (GMC GMP) and mental illness, which needs to be understood.

Table 11.1 Mental illness and professionalism

Relationships between health and professional practice	
Health problem might affect insight and ability to deliver safe care.	Depression, dementia, psychosis all can cause cognitive impairment. Mental health conditions such as depression, anxiety or bipolar disorder can impact cognitive functions such as decision-making, memory and concentration. In a medical setting, impaired cognitive abilities could lead to diagnosis, treatment or patient management errors.
Health problem might involve illegal or unprofessional activity, such as theft, self-prescribing.	Use of drugs such as strong opiates, stimulants and cannabis will need to involve the doctor engaging in illegal activities.
Health problem might be caused by a performance issue.	Depression or anxiety leading to inappropriate behaviour such as shouting or being abusive in the workplace.
Health problem might lead to misconduct.	Depression leading to shoplifting or drink-driving.
Health problem might require close supervision which can only be effectively done through the regulator.	Monitoring for drug or alcohol might not be possible in most workplaces and as such just arranging them might create disruption and additional costs for the employer.

(Continued)

Table 11.1 (*Continued*)	
Relationships between health and professional practice	
Complaint.	Might lead to a doctor becoming depressed or worsen a pre-existing mental illness.
Mental illness might be incompatible with practising as a doctor.	Dementia. Acute or untreated psychosis.
Poor performance can be amplified by mental illness.	A doctor who is struggling at work and making errors or not able to make decisions might become mentally unwell due to critical comments. This might then lead to anxiety and further performance issues.

INVOLVING THE REGULATOR?

Every doctor in the UK is bound to follow the GMC GMP, which sets out the requirements. Dentists must follow the requirements of the General Dental Council and other professional groups by the standards and requirements set out by their regulatory body.

REFER OR NOT REFER?

Concerning ill health, the GMC advise that (GMP 2024):

> *If you know or suspect that you have a serious condition that you could pass on to patients, or if your judgement or performance could be affected by a condition or its treatment, you must consult a suitably qualified colleague. You must follow their advice about any changes to your practice they consider necessary. You must not rely on your assessment of the risk to patients.*

- For details, refer to: *https://www.gmc-uk.org/professional-standards/professional-standards-for-doctors/good-medical-practice*

Deciding to refer or to encourage the doctor to refer themselves (and follow-up on this advice to ensure it is acted upon) is sometimes very difficult. This is why, wherever possible, it should be a team decision. The treating clinician must weigh *all* factors, including the regulatory requirements and issue/s relating to the potential risk they pose to their patients, employers or themselves. If the doctor is not working and, as such, not placing their patients at risk or is following specific advice from their treating team, then the decision need not be rushed. It is better to allow the sick doctor to get better (for example, to be admitted for drug/alcohol rehabilitation or treated with antidepressants) than to risk their psychological health worsening and even driving the sick doctor over the edge by having to engage with regulatory issues when unwell.

The GMC (2018) has issued guidance on what it expects to consider when determining whether a doctor needs to come to their attention irrespective of any underlying health problem, see:

- *https://www.gmc-uk.org/registration-and-licensing/join-the-register/what-to-tell-us-when-you-apply-guide/health-concerns-affecting-study-and-practice*

These include the following:

- Where there is a significant performance or conduct issue.
- Where the doctor has been convicted or cautioned.
- Where the doctor needs to follow the advice of a treating doctor or appears to need more insight.

Not all health and performance issues need to be investigated by the GMC or lead to a sanction. In some cases, it may be possible to address the allegation of misconduct or poor performance by dealing solely with the health problem and without taking specific action about the misconduct or performance issue.

They advise that three factors must be present for this to be the case.

1. Cogent evidence that a doctor's health is linked to the allegation of misconduct or poor performance.

   and

2. Where the doctor has a pre-existing health condition that poses a risk to their medical practice, there must be evidence that a doctor has taken steps to minimise the reoccurrence of any risks posed by their health, e.g., compliance with treatment. Where the incident happened at the onset of a condition or despite compliance with treatment, this will be regarded as a mitigating factor.

   and

3. Evidence that the allegations of misconduct or poor performance are at the lower end of the spectrum of matters that usually require action to protect patients or confidence in the medical profession.

As a result of these three factors, there must be no realistic prospect of establishing that a doctor's fitness to practise (FtP) is impaired because of the alleged misconduct and performance, and as such, the doctor can be treated as a pure health case rather than as a multifactorial case involving health and misconduct and performance.

For all cases, there must be consideration of the following:

- The type and severity of the mental illness and whether it is unlikely to affect a doctor's FtP or pose a risk to patients.

- There is no evidence that mental illness has significantly impacted performance or conduct.

- Evidence that the doctor has insight.

- The doctor receives appropriate support or treatment, or local employers/ supervisors are aware of the issues and can provide help.

- The doctor is in stable, long-term work or training or works only in appropriately supervised environments.

- Where necessary, the doctor has agreed to restrict their working practices in line with any advice given.

- If necessary, the doctor is not working.

- There is no relevant other FtP issues or significant history.

Examples of health affecting fitness to practise (FtP)

The following examples are based on cases from the GMC website. They are typical of doctors where a health issue might affect their FtP (and remember, placing the profession into disrepute is considered a FtP problem).

- *A doctor was cautioned by the police for possession of a Class B drug. A health assessment undertaken by the regulator finds that he uses cannabis regularly to control an anxiety disorder.*

This case is typical of those involving drug use and might include cannabis or amphetamines. Having been cautioned, the doctor is (or should ensure they are) made known to the UK regulator – caution is a formal warning given to a person who has admitted an offence. If the person refuses the caution, they will usually be prosecuted through the usual channels for the crime. Being cautioned is on the list of automatic referrals, and even if the police fail to do so, the practitioner must. However, other than being on their record, it is unlikely that the regulator will take any action, especially if the doctor has stopped using the drug/s in question and sought or is seeking help. The misconduct is closely linked to the doctor's health. It would not normally proceed to a full hearing, especially if the doctor has insight and there are no concerns about their clinical performance or risk to patients.

- *A doctor is causing concern at work, including being late for the clinic, arriving in a chaotic state and making a series of mistakes involving correspondence and record keeping, though no patient has been harmed. He also raised his voice at a colleague. He is asked to see his GP for a health assessment: The GP diagnoses depression, starts the doctor on treatment and advises that he take a brief time from work to help his recovery. The doctor accepts his health's impact on his work and discusses this with his senior colleague.*

Being late to a clinic due to depression or public transport delays irritates patients and colleagues, but repeated lateness is disruptive. This doctor has been making errors in his correspondence but poses little risk to his patients. By seeking and adhering to the advice of his GP, there is no need for any regulatory or disciplinary involvement.

- *A doctor receives a caution for shoplifting a few small items. Following the offence, the doctor seeks help from his GP, who diagnoses depression due to a series of life events (including her mother's death and an abusive relationship). The doctor is given a suspended sentence and asked to complete community service.*

This is an unfortunate case, as the doctor now has a criminal record. She cited shame and fear when asked why she did not seek help. The doctor will likely be able to work again, though given the legal sanction she received, she would automatically be referred by the Registrar to an MPTS hearing.

GMC HEALTH PROCEDURES

Investigations into a doctor's FtP might start in response to the doctor's disclosure or through contact from their employer, a member of the public or a patient. The police will often disclose any substance-related caution or conviction to the GMC. Any conviction or caution received anywhere in the world must be disclosed by the doctor in question, irrespective of the reason.

A GMC health investigation will start with assessments by two GMC-appointed psychiatrists. The GMC specifically asks the psychiatrist to provide a written opinion on a doctor's FtP by asking the psychiatrist to comment on whether:

a. The doctor is fit to practise without restriction

b. The doctor is not fit to practise or

c. The doctor is not fit to practise except on a limited basis or

d. The doctor is not fit to practise except under medical supervision or

e. The doctor is not fit to practise except on a limited basis and under medical supervision or

f. The doctor suffers from a recurring or episodic condition which, although in remission at the time of the assessment, may be expected in future to render her unfit to practise or unfit to practise except on a limited basis or under medical supervision or both

OUTCOME OF GMC INVESTIGATIONS

Depending on the outcome, the doctor may offer to agree to voluntary undertakings on their registration.

BOX 11.2: Summary of GMC processes

GMC provisional enquiries are limited enquiries into cases unlikely to reach the GMC's threshold for impairment of fitness to practise (FtP). The GMC obtains relevant information, which may include obtaining medical records, investigation reports, comments from the doctor concerned and an independent clinical view of the concerns. It will then decide if the case can be closed or whether it should be sent through to the FtP investigations procedure. A doctor should seek advice if they are subject to a provisional enquiry before providing comments about the concerns. Providing comments can be very helpful at this stage as the GMC will not usually refer to a full investigation if they are satisfied that there is no risk to patients arising from the concern and, where appropriate, that the doctor has taken steps to avoid repetition of a mistake and shown insight.

At any point during a GMC investigation, if there are serious concerns about the safety of patients or others, a doctor may be referred to an Interim Orders Tribunal that considers whether any action should be taken on a doctor's registration whilst the substantive investigation is ongoing. This could result in suspension or conditions.

Where a concern reaches the threshold for a **full GMC fitness-to-practice investigation**, the doctor will receive what is known as a Rule 4 letter with a copy of the complaint. Whilst a doctor can respond at this stage, they should seek advice from their MDO or solicitor before doing so. The GMC will investigate and, at this stage, can order an assessment of performance, knowledge of English or a health assessment.

If, after initial investigation, the GMC considers that there may be a case to answer, the doctor will receive a Rule 7 letter, which sets out the allegations and gives the doctor 28 days to respond. As for Preliminary Enquiries and Rule 4 letters, legal advice and assistance are recommended at this stage.

At the end of the investigation, the GMC Case Examiners will consider all the evidence provided and may conclude the case with no action, a letter of advice, give a warning, invite the doctor to accept undertakings or refer to an FtP tribunal.

FtP tribunals are managed by the Medical Practitioners Tribunal Service (MPTS). It may take several months before the hearing takes place, during which time the GMC will continue investigations and may seek expert evidence. The doctor's legal representatives may also seek expert evidence.

The outcomes include no action, undertakings, conditions, suspension or erasure.

The undertakings are essentially an assurance that the doctor has put in place a series of interventions to reassure the GMC that they are safe to practise until a time is reached for a fuller assessment or when the GMC is satisfied that the doctor is fit to practise with no restrictions. Undertakings are agreements between the GMC and a doctor about the doctor's future practice. Undertakings might stop a doctor from doing certain things (such as issuing certain medicines or working alone) or commit a doctor to only working while supervised. Whilst voluntary, a doctor is wise to accept them.

Conditions of practice may be imposed on a doctor's registration. A condition is a doctor's registration restriction, so they must wholly comply with it. Conditions can be placed on a doctor's registration before a full hearing, for example, by an Interim Orders Tribunal (IOT). Conditions may include supervision by a GMC-appointed doctor, which offers a supportive framework for recovery. Conditions of practice that are imposed might be minimally intrusive on a doctor's practice or very stringent, causing difficulty for a doctor. Conditions for doctors investigated for substance misuse almost always include abstinence from drugs and alcohol and an agreement to comply with arrangements for the announced or unannounced testing for the recent and long-term ingestion of alcohol or other drugs. The conditions might also include regular attendance at a support group or counselling service, e.g., Alcoholics Anonymous/Narcotics Anonymous/the Doctors and Dentists Group/any other support group/individual alcohol/drug counselling, providing the GMC evidence of attendance on request. Patients cannot be asked to attend Practitioner Health as part of their conditions or undertakings.

Failure to comply can lead to significant suspension if a doctor is deliberate or reckless in breaching the conditions.

It is important for the doctor to seek legal advice before agreeing to undertakings or conditions as some requirements might be difficult or even impossible to adhere to. For example, the employer cannot always provide mandated workplace supervision and workplace testing.

In 2015, research was carried out for the GMC into the impact of their sanctions on doctors, with the results showing that the sanctions had a major effect on doctors' future ability to work beyond the actual (sometimes short) sanction period. The research involved interviewing doctors who had received a sanction between 2006 and 2013, see:

- *https://www.gmc-uk.org/-/media/documents/The_effects_of_restrictions_or_warnings_research_report_FINAL.pdf_63538542.pdf*

Even the mildest response, **a warning**, had a lasting adverse impact.

A warning can be issued when a doctor's conduct or performance is found to be seriously below expected standards but not such that restrictions to their practice are warranted. Instead, it is intended as a guidance tool for doctors to improve their future practice.

Many doctors who received warnings were subsequently unable to return to work. Employers responded to warnings in diverse ways. In some cases, they ignored the warning, while at the opposite end of the spectrum, receiving a warning led to the termination of the doctor's employment relationship.

Many interviewed doctors found the **undertakings** and **conditions** impractical, making remediation an unattainable goal. As a result, the doctors' shortcomings often led to the termination of their medical practice and careers. Restrictions on medical practice are more likely to result in successful remediation in health-related cases than cases involving performance or misconduct. Several reasons contribute to this trend. One key factor is that doctors facing health issues are generally more receptive to and engaged with the imposed restrictions, unlike their counterparts in performance or misconduct cases. Additionally, colleagues and employers tend to support doctors with health-related undertakings and conditions more than those dealing with performance or misconduct issues. Nevertheless, almost a quarter of doctors with undertakings or conditions interviewed in this study could no longer work as a doctor.

Following an FtP hearing, the doctor might receive a service sanction, that is, a period of suspension or have their licence to practise removed (erasure).

Medical Practitioners Tribunal Service (MPTS)

The FtP hearing is a three-stage process:

1. **Fact-finding:** On the balance of probabilities (the civil standard of proof).

2. Decision on whether the doctor is impaired because the facts found proved.

3. If so, whether any action should be taken against the doctor's registration.

If the FtP tribunal decides to take no action against the doctor's registration, but there has been a significant departure from the standards in GMP, it may issue a warning.

After an IOT hearing or FtP tribunal, the document recording the decisions (the determination) is available to the public on the MPTS website.

The doctor's health information is redacted.

In February 2018, the GMC introduced time limits for how long historical sanctions and undertakings on a doctor's registration are published on the medical register. Previously, all sanctions and undertakings (excluding warnings) were published for five years but remained on GMC records indefinitely and could be disclosed to employers. They have now moved to two years published but remain on records and disclosable indefinitely so this section needs amending. The new time limits will vary according to the action taken, whether the doctor remains registered and whether the fitness-to-practise issues relate solely to the doctor's health.

The GMC have moved move to a new publication limit of two years for warnings – one year on the 'Doctor Details' page and one year on the 'History' page of the doctor's record. This will not be applied retrospectively. They will continue to disclose warnings to current employers indefinitely.

The GMC seeks to balance the need to be transparent and open with the public and its duty to be fair to the doctor.

Reasons for sanctions by the regulator

Most of the suspension or erasure cases arise from an incident in a doctor's working life, with only a few cases relating to a doctor's personal life. The latter has to be very serious and more likely to result from a criminal offence.

Overall, the most common type of case was dishonesty. GMP (2013) states that doctors must 'be honest and open and act with integrity'. Thus, dishonest conduct constitutes a serious departure from the fundamental tenets of GMP and the standards expected of a doctor. This is taken very seriously by Medical Practitioners Tribunal Service (MPTS) panels. The second most common type of case was inappropriate relations with patients and colleagues, but most frequently with patients. The third most common type of case was clinical issues, although a further proportion of cases involved dishonesty and clinical issues.

Most doctors who receive a severe sanction (suspension or erasure) by the GMC do not receive them for a health issue alone. The sanction is instead related to an issue in a doctor's working life (such as dishonesty, inappropriate relationships with patients or severe clinical errors).

The most common health reasons a doctor might be involved with the regulator are criminal charges relating to drug or alcohol (drink-driving) dependence. At Practitioner Health, addiction drug or alcohol misuse accounts for nearly half of all cases involving doctors in regulatory proceedings.

It is important to stress that most doctors with mental illness can present for care, receive treatment, get better and return to work without involving anyone other than their medical team. Doctors with serious mental illnesses, such as alcohol dependence, bipolar disorder or other psychotic conditions, do not necessarily need to involve the medical regulator. The mental health impact of being investigated by the regulator will be discussed later in this handbook.

REPORT WRITING

As a clinician involved in the care of a mentally ill health professional, the need to write a formal report often comes up. It might be a simple letter to an employer or a more formal report to a solicitor or regulator. It is always important to gain consent from the health professional before writing anything and to send draft versions of the correspondence to them to ensure the details are accurate and fair before disclosure to the requestor (GMC, *Good Medical Practice* deals with this paras 88–89 [https://www.gmc-uk.org/-/media/documents/gmp-2024-final---english_pdf-102607294.pdf]).

A report from an expert witness and a report from a treating clinician serve distinct purposes and come from different perspectives in the legal and medical fields. The key differences between the two are discussed below.

Role and relationship with the patient

Expert Witness: An expert witness is typically not involved in the direct care or treatment of the individual involved in the legal case. They are brought in to provide objective and impartial opinions based on their expertise and knowledge. They have no prior therapeutic relationship with the patient or client involved in the case.

Treating Clinician: A treating clinician is a healthcare professional (e.g., doctor, therapist, psychologist) who has an ongoing and direct therapeutic relationship with the patient. They are responsible for providing treatment and care to the patient and may have confidential patient-provider privileges.

Purpose

What objective do you and your patient hope to achieve with the letter? Given their current emotional state, is the letter in your patient's best interests? Talk with your patient about the potential benefits and risks, including issues around privacy and confidentiality.

Expert Witness: The primary purpose of an expert witness report is to offer an independent, objective and professional opinion in legal proceedings. The expert's report aims to help the court or the parties involved understand complex medical or psychological issues and provide clarity on specific aspects of the case.

Treating Clinician: A report from a treating clinician is created as part of the standard medical or therapeutic process. It is focused on the patient's diagnosis, treatment, progress and therapeutic recommendations. The treating clinician's report is primarily for the benefit of the patient's care and may not be shared in legal proceedings unless consent is given or under exceptional circumstances.

Objectivity

Ahead of agreeing to write any report, ask if you are qualified to write it. If you are not comfortable with the request, ask yourself why not? If it's anxiety or inexperience, collaborating with a colleague might help. On the other hand, if it's because of a conflict of interest or because you haven't seen the patient in several years, you probably want to decline the request.

Expert Witness: An expert witness is expected to maintain objectivity and impartiality. Their opinion should be based solely on their professional expertise and not influenced by any personal or therapeutic relationship with the patient.

Treating Clinician: A treating clinician is directly involved in the patient's care and may have a therapeutic relationship with them. This relationship can potentially impact the clinician's objectivity, as they focus on providing their patient the best care.

Confidentiality

Expert Witness: An expert witness does not typically have a therapeutic relationship with the patient and is not bound by the same confidentiality rules as a treating clinician. Their primary responsibility is to provide accurate information to the court.

Treating Clinician: Treating clinicians are bound by patient-provider confidentiality, and they usually must seek the patient's consent before sharing any medical or psychological information with third parties, including in legal proceedings.

In summary, the key distinctions between a report from an expert witness and a report from a treating clinician lie in their roles, the nature of their relationship with the patient, their objectives and their obligations regarding objectivity and confidentiality. An expert witness provides an impartial opinion in a legal context, while a treating clinician's report focuses on the patient's care and treatment.

When writing the report, consider the following

STRUCTURE

In some cases, the requesting agency provides a detailed list of what your letter should include. However, in most situations, you will need to use your clinical judgement as to what constitutes 'need-to-know' information. For example, is the letter's purpose to help the patient work-related adjustments or a change in their training programme? Or is it to explain why a relapse might have occurred and what mitigating factors the employer might want to take into account? Make sure to frame any recommendations as your professional opinion.

Before starting work on a report, understand why you are writing it (expert, treating clinician, factual details). Ideally, have a written request (instruction) from a solicitor, coroner or whoever has asked you to provide the report. They may wish you to follow a structure using their headings.

Using the written request this way will help your report stay focused on what has been requested.

Example structure: Amplify or reduce as appropriate:

Introduction: Who requested this report? What is your role?

Interview: History of current difficulties; personal history; employment, substance misuse and conviction histories; physical and mental health histories.

Mental state examination.

Special investigations, if any.

Information from the papers (may include medical records).

The summary, including diagnosis, may include a comment about strengths and vulnerabilities.

Conclusions and answers to specific questions in the request.

LENGTH

Aim for a short report which is to the point. Include enough of the history (and any examinations – mental state examination? blood tests?) so that it is clear to the reader why you have come to your conclusions.

OPINIONS IN YOUR CONCLUSION

Use words carefully. For example, avoid absolutes, comment positively on the patient's strengths, explain your conclusions and ensure your opinion is balanced. Would the report be fair if the conclusions were tested in a legal forum? Sleep on the finished report and reread it the next day.

STATEMENT OF TRUTH

This is not necessary for reports to regulators or other clinicians.

Reports for courts must contain the following statement, which goes in above the signature:

> *I confirm that I have made clear which facts and matters referred to in this report are within my knowledge and which are not. Those that are within my knowledge I confirm to be true. The opinions I have expressed represent my true and complete professional opinions on the matters to which they refers.*

12

Confidentiality and information sharing

Questions about the boundaries of **confidentiality** are common when consulting with doctors, and it is wise to establish ground rules as early as possible, particularly around information sharing. This can be done through the material on the service's website or at the start of the consultation. Confidentiality is never absolute. There is a duty to disclose information in certain circumstances, such as safeguarding and where there is a risk of harm to a member of the public (or in the case of doctors, their patients), or to do so would be in the public interest.

The GMC states in their confidentiality guidance:

> If a patient objects to personal information being shared for their care, you should not disclose the information unless it would be justified in the public interest or is of overall benefit to a patient who cannot make the decision...You should explain to the patient the potential consequences of a decision not to allow personal information to be shared with others who are providing their care. It would be best to consider whether any compromise could be reached with the patient. If, after discussion, a patient who can make the decision still objects to disclosing personal information that you are convinced is essential to provide safe care, you should explain that you cannot refer them or otherwise arrange for their treatment without disclosing that information.
>
> **[Regulation 30]**

(https://www.gmc-uk.org/ethical-guidance/ethical-guidance-for-doctors/ confidentiality/using-and-disclosing-patient-information-for-direct-care)

It might be helpful to start the consultation with something along these lines:

Thank you for coming to see me. To say a few things before we get going: everything you tell me is confidential to the service unless I must disclose it. For example, if I am apprehensive about your safety or that of the patients you are treating, I might need to act without asking your permission. But be reassured that this is rare, and I will not disclose any details verbally or in writing without your consent. So.... how can I help?

INFORMATION SHARING

When sharing information, the Caldicott principles should be followed to ensure that information identifying a patient is protected and only used when appropriate.

The Caldicott principles

PRINCIPLE 1: JUSTIFY THE PURPOSE(S) FOR USING CONFIDENTIAL INFORMATION

Every proposed use or transfer of personal confidential data within or from an organisation should be clearly defined, scrutinised and documented, with continuing services regularly reviewed, by an appropriate guardian.

PRINCIPLE 2: DON'T USE PERSONAL CONFIDENTIAL DATA UNLESS IT IS NECESSARY

Personal confidential data items should only be included if it is essential for that flow's specified purpose(s). The need for identifying patients should be considered at each stage of satisfying the purpose(s).

PRINCIPLE 3: USE THE MINIMUM NECESSARY PERSONAL CONFIDENTIAL DATA

Where the use of personal confidential data is essential, the inclusion of each item of data should be considered and justified so that the minimum amount of personal confidential data is transferred or accessible as necessary for a given function to be carried out.

PRINCIPLE 4: ACCESS TO PERSONAL CONFIDENTIAL DATA SHOULD BE ON A STRICT NEED-TO-KNOW BASIS

Only those individuals who need access to personal confidential data should have access to it, and they should only have access to the items they need to see. This may mean introducing access controls or splitting data flows where one data flow is used for several purposes.

PRINCIPLE 5: EVERYONE WITH ACCESS TO PERSONAL CONFIDENTIAL DATA SHOULD BE AWARE OF THEIR RESPONSIBILITIES

Action should be taken to ensure that those handling personal confidential data – both clinical and non-clinical staff – are fully aware of their responsibilities and obligations to respect patient confidentiality.

PRINCIPLE 6: COMPLY WITH THE LAW

Every use of personal confidential data must be lawful. Someone in each organisation handling personal confidential data should be responsible for ensuring that the organisation complies with legal requirements.

PRINCIPLE 7: THE DUTY TO SHARE INFORMATION CAN BE AS CRUCIAL AS PROTECTING PATIENT CONFIDENTIALITY

Health and social care professionals should have the confidence to share information in the best interests of their patients within the framework set out by these principles. They should be supported by the policies of their employers, regulators and professional bodies.

Sharing information is part of everyday teamwork, and unless the practitioner-patient has explicitly asked that some team members not access their records or be part of any discussions (for example, when they have a very close personal or professional relationship), then sharing should be expected as part of routine care.

There are circumstances where it would be necessary (and essential) to share information with the practitioner–patient's general practitioner or other health professional involved in their care.

These are as follows:

- Concern about the level of risk to themselves or others and where this cannot be managed alone.
- The patient's care needs to be transferred to local services, such as an outreach team, for in-patient care or day-care services not otherwise accessible by the service.
- Ongoing prescribing requirements include long-term prescribing of anti depressants, anxiolytics or medicines required for alcohol and drug maintenance.
- Where there are safeguarding concerns about dependents or other adults.
- There are concerns that the patient is unstable with a severe mental condition that might require GP/community intervention.
- Where required by law.

13

Management of mental illness

When thinking about burnout, compassion fatigue, depression, anxiety or any mental illness, what is important is recognising when one can go on no longer, when negative attitudes turn to loss of compassion and when one's behaviour changes to the detriment (such as becoming irritable, withdrawing from social events and so on).

MANAGEMENT OF BURNOUT, DEPRESSION AND ANXIETY

Think of the following case scenario:

Richard is a senior partner in a six-partner GP practice. The previous senior partner retired 12 months ago, and he took over as the longest-serving doctor in the practice. Since then, he reports that the partnership is in free fall. The practice manager has come to him saying she has had enough. She is looking to leave as soon as she can find another job. One partner is already working on her notice, and the younger partners want to work part-time as they feel their mental health cannot cope with the workload.

This has been affecting his health for several months. He used to love work but now dreads going in, often needing to spend up to 30 minutes in his car, stationary in the car park at work, before having the energy to go in and face the day. He avoids all his partners whenever possible and spends most of his time in his room. He admits to drinking every night. He used only to drink one or two evenings per week but now drinks up to a bottle of wine four to five nights weekly. He knows this is too much but feels he needs that 'quick fix' after a busy day. His sleep is poor; he has gained weight, finds it difficult to make decisions and is becoming increasingly forgetful. He has considered suicide but does not want to die, instead just wanting 'it all to go away'. He has not confided in his wife as she is recovering from an operation, nor has he sought support from his children as one is currently doing their finals at medical school, and the other is about to have her first baby.

DOI: 10.1201/9781003391500-13

He feels responsible for keeping his 'chin up' for his wife's benefit and supporting his children emotionally and financially. He feels very responsible for the state of the practice, as he believes all the issues started when he took over. Life has become hopeless.

QUESTIONS

- *Is Richard suffering from a mental illness? If so, what might this be?*

- *What is your formulation of his current situation?*

- *Who might you manage him?*

- *What local support might you suggest?*

IDENTIFICATION OF BURNOUT

Anyone working close to human suffering will develop some aspects of burnout at some point in their career. Just as ageing results from a successful healthcare system, burnout is the inevitable consequence of caring. Emotional depletion, negative attitudes towards patients and the feeling that we cannot achieve more are not uncommon and hopefully fleeting symptoms.

One of the handbook authors, CG, has devised simple questions to identify burnout. It is based on the CAGE questionnaire used in screening for alcohol misuse, though the acronym fits for identifying burnout.

1. Has anyone close to you asked you to Cut down on your work?

2. Have you recently become Angry or resentful about your work or patients?

3. Do you feel Guilty that you are not spending enough time with your friends, family, or yourself?

4. Do you find yourself becoming increasingly Emotional, for example, crying, getting angry, shouting, or feeling tense for no apparent reason?

When managing burnout, since it is an occupational disease, the best place to start in 'treatment' is to address the environment in which doctors work. Whilst this might not be in the treating clinician's gift, empathising with the doctor and deflecting responsibility for their well-being into their workplace (rather than themselves) can help gain a sense of agency. Everyone performs better in environments with good internal communication systems, where we feel supported by management, where there are opportunities for professional development and where leaders are competent.

On the other hand, environments where excessive workload, long work hours, fatigue, intense emotional interactions, restricted autonomy and constant structural and organisational changes become the norm lead to an increased risk of burnout.[73] The psychologist Howard Schwartz distinguished between two types of organisations: clockwork (*running smoothly, cooperative, low anxiety*) or snake pit (*everything is falling apart, high-stress levels, little pleasure or joy at work*).[74] Organisations with more 'snake pit' features are likely to create risks for burnout. This means that the staff is the most significant threat in underfunded, understaffed environments that demand high productivity at all costs.

The most important interventions, therefore, must be targeted at addressing workplace stressors.[75] These include work pressure, resources (time, people and finances) and creating opportunities for teamwork. On a larger scale, it means amending external factors, such as regulatory requirements, political influences and media pressures, all contributing to chronic workplace distress.[76] Treating burnout as a public health crisis might mean we use the same prevention strategies as with any other threat to the public's health.

IDENTIFICATION OF DEPRESSION

Identifying depression can be challenging, as its symptoms can overlap with other mental health issues, including physical illnesses. However, there are common signs and symptoms to look out for, which can indicate that someone might be experiencing depression.

These symptoms include:

- **Persistent sadness or low mood:** Feeling consistently sad, hopeless, or empty.

- **Loss of interest or pleasure:** Losing interest in activities and hobbies that were once enjoyable.

- **Changes in appetite or weight:** Significant changes in eating habits, leading to weight gain or loss.

- **Sleep disturbances:** Experiencing insomnia (difficulty falling asleep or staying asleep) or hypersomnia (excessive sleeping).

- **Fatigue and decreased energy:** Feeling tired and lacking the energy to perform daily tasks.

- **Feelings of worthlessness or guilt:** Frequent self-criticism, feelings of guilt and a negative self-image.

- **Difficulty concentrating or making decisions:** Struggling with focus, memory and decision-making.

- **Irritability or restlessness:** Feeling easily annoyed or agitated.

- **Physical symptoms:** Unexplained aches, pains and digestive problems.

- **Social withdrawal:** Isolating oneself from friends and family, avoiding social interactions.

- **Recurrent thoughts of death or suicide:** Thinking about death or wanting to die.

TREATMENT

Most clinical interventions involve mindfulness, behavioural treatment, mentoring, coaching, or addressing personal coping strategies[77] and can include:

- Counselling to empower a doctor's sense of agency.

- Mindfulness to develop a keen awareness and relaxation.

- Cognitive behavioural therapy can help bring awareness to various thinking errors, including emotional reasoning.

- Stress management techniques.

- Assertiveness training: Learning to say 'no' without fear of repercussion.

- Professional coaching which enhances the sense of efficacy and self-determination by strengthening professional skills and using a behavioural approach to tackle negative inner dialogue.

- Signposting to a peer support group.

- Exam support for doctors in training.

Work-related adjustments that could be suggested to the doctor include the following:

- Reducing hours to less than full-time.

- Re-organising a work rota to accommodate sleep deprivation and recovery time.

- Normalise and formalise breaks to be taken in a work schedule.

- Compassionate leadership principles to fully understand the causes of distress and how to reduce the impact of stressors.

- Peer support groups: Emotional support for the emotional demands.

MANAGEMENT OF ADDICTION

This section will explore how to manage a patient with drug or alcohol addiction. The first stage is to understand when the patient is ready to change their habits, as discussed below. When reading this chapter, think of the following case scenario:

John is a 42-year-old GP, a new partner in a large practice.

Stage 1. At the end of his initial assessment

His appraiser suggested he self-refer to Practitioner Health after it came to light locally that he had been self-prescribing tramadol, under practice patient identities. A fellow partner picked this up. He had begun using tramadol following knee surgery approximately 18 months ago. He is currently using 150 mg daily, three times a day. He described himself as being a lifelong worrier and poor sleep for 'as long as I can remember', and that the tramadol helps him get some sleep. He is a father to two young children, and his wife is also a GP in another local practice. He has not told his wife at the time of assessment.

Ever since, medical school he has worried about complaints, mistakes and being 'found out'. There has also been a merger with a neighbouring failing practice and a recent CQC visit. He reports a troubled childhood with parents who demanded perfection and obedience, and he was punished if he did not achieve.

At assessment, you find him to be depressed with significant features of anxiety, and this may well have been the case for several years. He describes a feeling of 'being on a knife edge' since NHS England had been in touch. He has not been formally suspended by either his practice or NHSE. He wants it all to go away and get back to work. He's already written to all his colleagues in the practice and apologised, and 'just wants to get back to normal ASAP'.

Points to consider:

- *What do you and the patient need to discuss before he leaves?*

- *Any thoughts on his risk and how this could be managed?*

- *Who else might we involve? Why and when?*

- *From a mental health/addiction point of view, what is the treatment priority?*

- *What would you be advising about work?*

Stage 2. Four weeks after initial assessment

After the last appointment, he told his wife, who was very angry, about his drug use and asked him to leave the house. He stayed in a hotel for two nights, and she then allowed him back. He has not worked in the last four weeks. He was never suspended from his practice and remains 'on leave'. He followed your advice and self-referred to the GMC. An interim orders panel at the GMC was convened within two weeks, and temporary conditions (involuntary restrictions) were placed on his practice. He is not allowed to prescribe opiates and must not work alone in his practice (other doctors must always be available for advice/support). He has yet to be assessed by the GMC and wants to return to work as soon as possible. In the last four weeks, he has attempted to stop the tramadol on two occasions without success and has more recently accepted your initial offer of starting substitution therapy, buprenorphine. Needing to take buprenorphine makes him feel 'like an addict', he said, and he wants to reduce and stop ASAP.

Whilst the buprenorphine effectively stops any physical withdrawal symptoms, he reports poor sleep, anxiety and low mood.

Points to consider:

- *How might we assist in the GMC process?*

- *How might we assist him in a timely return to work?*

- *What might the issues be with a GP versus a hospital Dr, as GP partners are typically self-employed, especially regarding return to work and occupational health support?*

- *What are your thoughts on people who have used drugs and who struggle to accept any associated labels or paths towards help?*

Stage 3. Three months following a return to work

Your patient has successfully returned to work on both buprenorphine and an antidepressant that was added later. They are working under GMC conditions set in the interim orders panel. NHS England has now reported the prescribing irregularities to the police. Your patient has been asked to attend an interview cautiously in two weeks. He is keen to stop the buprenorphine and is currently on a small dose.

Points to consider:

- *What would your advice be around stopping buprenorphine, and do you have any suggestions on the timings of this?*

- *What advice might you offer regarding the police interview/process?*

- *Do you have any predictions of how this might affect his registration or ability to practise?*

What support might you offer or explore with this patient?

STAGES OF RECOVERY

A careful assessment can help determine what stage of preparedness they are to address their addiction.

Mary sat alone in her office; her tired eyes fixed on the half-empty whiskey bottle. She had once been a promising doctor, driven by a genuine desire to comfort those in need. But over time, the stress of her work had taken its toll. Long hours, sleepless nights and constant exposure to human suffering had chipped away at her resilience, leaving her vulnerable and seeking solace in the numbing embrace of alcohol.

She reached for the bottle, her hand trembling slightly. Her gaze shifted to the framed photograph on her desk – a picture of her younger self, clad in a crisp white coat, surrounded by colleagues who had long since moved on to greener pastures. They had found happiness, while Mary remained stuck in a cycle of self-destruction.

As she made her way home, she passed her ward; the smell of disinfectant and the cacophony of alarms and urgent voices intensified her anxiety. The pressure mounted, suffocating her and her hand involuntarily twitched, yearning for the familiar burn of alcohol that used to silence her fears.

At that moment, Mary recognised that her patients deserved better – a doctor who could provide the care they needed, unburdened by the destructive chains of addiction. She was determined to seek help. It was a small step towards healing.

In a moment of clarity, Mary gained insight into her problem and that she needed help. She has moved from the *pre-contemplation* to the *contemplation* stage of recovery. The psychologists Prochaska, DiClemente and Norcross[78] described the stages of change (called transtheoretical model, TTM), initially to help people stop smoking, but then expanded to other substance misuse.

The stages of change in the TTM are as follows:

1. **Precontemplation:** Individuals may be unaware of their problem. They may express resistance or denial when confronted with the need to change.

2. **Contemplation:** Individuals start considering the possibility of change. They may weigh the pros and cons though still experience ambivalence about changing their behaviour.

3. **Preparation:** Individuals may start making small steps towards change. This might be gathering information, setting goals and making plans to modify their behaviour.

4. **Action:** Individuals actively modify their behaviour, environment, or both to bring about change. This stage requires commitment, effort and the implementation of specific strategies or interventions.

5. **Maintenance:** Individuals enter the maintenance stage after successfully implementing the desired change. They work to sustain the behaviour change over time, preventing relapse and consolidating new habits.

6. **Termination:** In some versions of the TTM, a termination stage is included, where individuals have successfully stopped their problem behaviour and no longer feel tempted to return to it.

Throughout the stages, individuals may encounter challenges, relapses and setbacks. The model recognises that progress is only sometimes linear and that individuals may move back and forth between stages. It emphasises the importance of self-efficacy, decisional balance (weighing the benefits and costs of change) and supportive environments in facilitating successful behaviour change.

The **Prochaska, DiClemente and Norcross Models** have influenced interventions to promote health behaviour, addiction recovery and other personal transformations. It underscores the need for tailored approaches addressing an individual's specific readiness stage and acknowledges the complexity of the process (Figure 13.1).

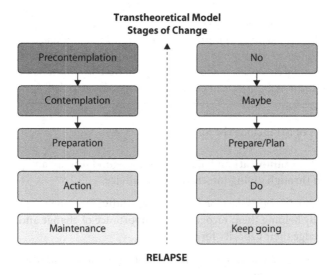

Figure 13.1 Transtheoretical model.

The stages can last from months to years, depending on the severity of the addiction and the individual's experience. For some, it can take only a few months of abstinence to reach the point where they don't return to their addictive behaviour. However, for most, a commitment of two to five years is necessary to break the habit and solidify change.

OVERCOMING AMBIVALENCE TO CHANGE

Managing doctors with addiction requires a multifaceted and compassionate approach, prioritising the individual's well-being and patients' safety. The mainstay of treatment is a focus on abstinence, though controlled drinking for alcohol addiction and the prescribing of substitute medication can be helpful for some patients.

Achieving abstinence can be a hard and long struggle for many, with those finding it difficult often individuals who are reluctant to accept that they have a serious problem, leading to their tendency to cover up relapses under the guise of '*I don't have a serious problem*'. This can be understood as denial or a lack of insight. The addicted clinician maintains a facade that they are 'well', even when they continue drinking and using drugs and struggle with physical, psychological and social negative consequences – e.g., symptomatic alcohol-related liver disease, depression, relationship breakdown and homelessness.

MOTIVATIONAL INTERVIEWING

Motivational interviewing (MI) helps nudge the individual to gain insight, remove barriers and engage in treatment.[79]

> Motivational interviewing (MI) is defined as *collaborative, goal-oriented communication style with particular attention to the language of change. It is designed to strengthen personal motivation for and commitment to a specific goal by eliciting and exploring the person's reasons for change within an atmosphere of acceptance and compassion* (p. 29).

Key qualities of MI include the following:

- **Balanced communication:** Balancing being a good listener and providing direction through giving information and advice.
- **Empowerment:** MI is designed to empower individuals to make positive changes by helping them recognise the importance of change and acknowledge their capacity for change.
- **Respectful and curious approach:** MI promotes natural change and the individual's autonomy.
- **Equal partnership:** MI necessitates that the clinician engages with the patient as an equal partner in the conversation. Unsolicited advice, confrontation, instruction, direction, or warnings should be avoided.
- **Not imposing change:** MI is not a means to forcefully 'get people to change'. Instead, it is a collaborative and patient-centred approach.

MI is particularly beneficial in situations where:

- **Ambivalence exists:** When individuals are grappling with mixed feelings about change.
- **Low confidence:** When individuals doubt their ability to make changes.
- **Low desire:** When individuals are unsure about whether they want to change.
- **Low importance:** When the change's benefits and the current situation's disadvantages are unclear.

MI encompasses skills encapsulated by the acronym **OARS**, which involves skilfully attending to the language of change and facilitating the exchange of information:

- *Open questions:* Open questions elicit and explore the individual's experiences, perspectives and ideas. Evocative questions guide patients to reflect on the personal significance and feasibility of change. Information is often imparted within the framework of open questions using the

Elicit–Provide–Elicit structure, which begins by exploring the person's existing knowledge, seeks permission to share the practitioner's insights and then delves into the person's response.

- **Affirmation:** Affirming strengths, efforts and past achievements is crucial in nurturing the person's optimism and self-assurance in their capacity to effect change.

- **Reflections:** Rooted in attentive listening, aiming to understand what the individual conveys by restating, rephrasing, or making informed suppositions about their underlying messages.

- **Summarisation:** This ensures a shared understanding and reinforces points raised during the conversation.

Attending to change language: MI practitioners pay close attention to the language used regarding change. They identify expressions that either support change (change talk) or resist it (sustain talk). When appropriate, they encourage a shift from sustained talk towards change talk.

MAKING THE DIAGNOSIS OF ADDICTION

Mark stood in front of the bathroom mirror, his bloodshot eyes reflecting his exhaustion. He sighed heavily, burdened by a secret he couldn't escape. It would be another hard day at the hospital, and he was already late again. Mornings were terrible for him due to alcohol, which had become his coping mechanism.

The faint smell of alcohol clung to his breath, a constant reminder of his double life. He tried to hide the smell with extra strong mints. He had always prided himself on his professionalism, and the thought of jeopardising his reputation terrified him. He couldn't afford to lose the trust of his patients or colleagues or his income.

Leaving the bathroom, he went to his office, heart pounding with guilt and desperation. With trembling hands, he retrieved a small flask from his coat pocket, discreetly pouring a measure of whiskey into his coffee cup. Careful not to draw attention, he took a quick sip, feeling momentary relief from the weight on his shoulders.

Throughout the day, Mark skilfully concealed his struggle behind a façade of competence. He diagnosed patients, prescribed medications, and carried out procedures while battling his demons secretly. It was a dangerous dance, a hidden addiction threatening to undo everything he had worked so hard to achieve.

Identifying alcohol (or drug) dependence can be difficult, especially when the doctor denies or tries to cover up their use. There are few diagnostic signs for drug/alcohol use, such as apparent intoxication, needle marks and smell of alcohol, but most signs of alcohol dependence are non-specific. Certain behaviours have a high index of suspicion that drug or alcohol addiction might be the underlying issue. For example, driving under the influence of alcohol.

Some non-specific signs and symptoms that might raise concerns include the following:

- Observable shifts in behaviour, such as increased irritability, mood swings or unexplained aggression.
- Frequent headaches, unexplained weight loss or gain, changes in appetite, unsteady gait, alcoholic smell on breath, tremors, or bloodshot eyes.
- Disregard personal grooming, wearing dishevelled clothes or neglecting personal hygiene.
- Withdrawing from family, friends and social activities that were previously enjoyed.
- Work performance declines, such as missed appointments, increased errors, or a lack of attention to detail.
- Sudden financial problems include frequent borrowing, requesting advances or unpaid bills.
- Engaging in secretive or suspicious activities, such as hiding substances or being evasive about one's whereabouts.
- Frequent conflicts or strained relationships with colleagues, friends, or family members.
- Involvement in legal issues related to substance use, such as drink-driving arrests or drug-related offences.
- Unexplained or recurring health issues (especially hypertension, gastritis, gout), frequent illnesses or a decline in overall health.

It is important to remember that these are non-specific and do not necessarily guarantee the presence of a substance-use disorder.

Some indicators suggest a substance use problem. These include mood swings; withdrawal from family, friends and leisure; spending more time at work and doing extra shifts; physical health problems such as weight loss and sick leave; unnecessary use of opioids with signing out increasing quantities; a consistent pattern of complaints and rumours; performance deterioration or significant change in working behaviour and other circumstantial evidence such as working alone, opting for irregular hours, volunteering to draw up drugs for others.

Most doctors with substance use disorders initially display symptoms outside the workplace rather than within it, usually for several years. They manage to hang on to work whilst everything else in their lives – their health, family, social life and self-esteem crumble.

There are some physical illnesses which suggest alcohol as a cause. These are:

- Hypertension
- Gastritis
- Depression

These within the same patient would indicate excess alcohol use as their cause until proven otherwise.

THE 'CAGE' QUESTIONNAIRE FOR ALCOHOL – SELF-ASSESSMENT TOOL[80]

This questionnaire is *not* designed to provide a diagnosis. It is, however, an easy-to-remember and a helpful screening tool.

A high score suggests the need for further and complete evaluation.

Scoring is 0 for 'no' and 1 for 'yes'. A total score of 2 or greater is considered indicative of an alcohol or drug problem.

1. Have you ever felt you should Cut down on your drinking?

2. Have people Annoyed you by criticising your drinking?

3. Have you felt bad or Guilty about your drinking?

4. Have you drunk alcohol first thing in the morning to steady your nerves? Or get rid of a hangover (Eye-opener)?

The Alcohol Use Disorders Identification Test (AUDIT) questionnaire is also useful. AUDIT is a 10-question alcohol harm screening tool. It was developed by the World Health Organisation (WHO) and modified for use in the UK and has been used in various health and social care settings. It is freely available:

- *https://assets.publishing.service.gov.uk/government/uploads/system/uploads/ attachment_data/file/1113175/Alcohol-use-disorders-identification-test-AUDIT_ for-print.pdf*

The Severity of Alcohol Dependence Questionnaire (SADQ) is a self-administered, 20-item questionnaire designed explicitly by the WHO to assess the severity of alcohol dependence in individuals who have been identified as having alcohol dependency. It aims to measure the level of dependence on alcohol by examining various aspects related to alcohol consumption and its impact on an individual's life.

The questionnaire covers a range of items assessing the physical and psychological symptoms, behavioural patterns and consequences of alcohol dependence. By self-reporting their experiences, individuals can provide valuable information that helps professionals gauge the severity of their alcohol dependency. It is free to download:

- *https://www.smartcjs.org.uk/wp-content/uploads/2015/07/SADQ.pdf*

Doctors who use drugs or alcohol stand out as different from other non-medical addicts in the nature and pattern of their use. For example, few use drugs daily and most use sporadically – when on holiday or off duty. It is unusual for them to use at work (especially early on in their addiction), though some do. Their pattern of use can be unique and related to their rota. So even when a doctor has alcohol dependency (as evidenced by, perhaps, craving, withdrawal, escalation of use or salience), they might 'only' *use* when not on duty or working the following day. This is much more akin to binge-drinking than the pattern of drinking we see in more typical alcohol dependence.

Doctors' use of illegal drugs should be considered problematic irrespective of the type of use, pattern or amounts. In the UK, using any illicit substance constitutes a fitness to practice issue, and whilst the doctor might not be dependent, their use is problematic.

The aim of the assessment

The main aims of the **assessment** are to:

- Obtain a drug and alcohol history, including route, quantity and frequency.
- Any previous treatment and its outcome.
- Address any physical health complications relating to use – injection site infections, lung, neurological, gastrointestinal and liver health.
- Try to determine the patient's readiness to change.
- Look for risky behaviours associated with/impacted by their addiction, including sexual health risks, personal safety risks, blood-borne virus exposure and vaccination status and overdoses.
- Establish Driving and Driving Vehicle Licencing Authority (DVLA) notification requirements.
- Jointly work through a management plan (short and longer term)
- Discuss whether the doctor needs to disclose themselves (or be declared) to the Regulator.
- Identify safeguarding risks to themselves and household members/ dependents, e.g., intoxicated when caring for vulnerable individuals, substances left out/not stored safely and strangers attending the house.
- Assess co-morbid mental health conditions, mental health assessment and suicide/homicide risk.

As a shorthand for assessing whether someone is dependent on the substance, it is sometimes helpful to explore the 3Cs:

- Control – or, more accurately, loss of control.

- Craving – and preoccupation with use.

- Consequences – of use despite the consequences.

This information is then used to formulate a management plan based on the individual's needs. It should be itself a therapeutic process. It can be one of the first instances of linking substance use/addictions to other problems experienced in their life. It is also an opportunity to objectively quantify the benefits and enhance their self-awareness.

DETOXIFICATION

In the main, addiction management is the same as any other non-medical patient. This means ensuring that risks are not taken when prescribing powerful psychotropic medications or undertaking community (home) detoxification.

Treatment's primary focus is abstinence from drugs and alcohol, which will necessitate stopping use (**detoxification**). Medication-assisted detoxification is frequently needed to prevent withdrawal symptoms and to provide a safe transition to a drug or alcohol-free state. For alcohol, this is either reducing the dose of diazepam or chlordiazepoxide together with thiamine. Dosing regimens are those found in standard medical formularies. For drug dependence, Practitioner Health typically uses reducing doses of buprenorphine – again in average amounts as in good practice guidelines.

It is helpful to use the established Clinical Guidelines on Drug Misuse and Dependence Update 2017 Independent Expert Working Group (2017) Drug misuse and dependence: UK guidelines on clinical management. London: Department of Health:

- *https://www.gov.uk/government/publications/drug-misuse-and-dependence-uk-guidelines-on-clinical-management*

Patients with low levels of opioid dependence, for example, secondary to over-the-counter or prescribed medication misuse, can be offered buprenorphine detoxification in the community setting.

Detoxification can take place in a community or residential setting. In Northern America, treatment is typically residential, and the patient is expected to complete a 12-week rehabilitation programme. For those engaged with Physician Health Programmes, 78% of addicted doctors entered residential treatment for at least 72 days. Ninety-five per cent of the programmes were 12-step in modality and abstinence focussed. Excepting antidepressants, medication played little part in treatment.

Other programmes, including patients attending NHS Practitioner Health, offer the patient a choice of whether to enter a residential or community-based detoxification and aftercare programme. NHS PH patients are given a choice based on their circumstances (for example, family responsibilities) rather than mandated, as in the North American PHPs, to undertake residential care. Where the residential option is chosen, this is for a 6-week (not the 12 weeks as in the USA) period. Outcomes amongst those who attended NHS Practitioner Health are similar, with around 80% of patients remaining abstinent at five-year follow-ups, irrespective of the treatment setting.[81–83]

WHEN TO REFER DOCTORS WITH SUBSTANCE MISUSE DISORDER TO THE REGULATOR (GMC OR GDC)

Doctors managing addiction patients are often concerned about whether they need to refer or strongly encourage their patients to disclose themselves to their Regulator. It is essential to spend some time discussing this, as often, the treating doctor rushes into disclosure when none is needed. There are some clear-cut requirements, such as following a criminal charge or caution. Any doctors charged or convicted of a drink or drug-related offence, including drink (or drug) driving, must refer themselves to the GMC or GDC. The police or Court usually does this, but the individual doctor must ensure that this disclosure has occurred; for most doctors who use alcohol or legally obtained drugs, the need to disclose is more nuanced and depends on various factors.

Whether or not to suggest **disclosure** depends on the following:

1. Where a patient might be placing their patients at risk?

2. Where, if still working, they are not engaging with treatment or adhering to our advice?

3. Where they continue to engage in illegal activities (including drug taking)?

Deciding whether or when to refer a practitioner–patient to their respective regulatory authority can pose a challenging dilemma for the treating clinician. In cases involving alcohol-related issues, it is feasible to provide support and treatment without requiring a referral unless certain circumstances apply. For instance, there would usually be no need to suggest a referral to the regulator where the doctor has not committed a criminal offence related to alcohol consumption and does not pose a risk to patient safety as they are following medical advice such as taking sick leave whilst receiving treatment.

On the other hand, where a doctor endangers others, including patients and the public, involving others with jurisdiction over the doctor might be essential. Take the case of Dr Charles Elswick (a fictional case), who was drinking half a bottle of vodka most evenings, though recently, this had increased with now drinking in the early mornings. He is a neurosurgeon. At his assessment, it was clear that he arrived at work intoxicated, often driving the five miles or so to work. He told his treating doctor this with an air of bravado. He tried to hide his use at work by sucking extra strong mints and eating onions. He did not want to stop working, especially as he had a lucrative private practice, which he did in the evenings. No matter what the treating clinician advised, he could not seem to understand the risk he posed to his patients (and to members of the public due to his drink-driving). The service had no option but to inform the doctor's occupational health physician, leading to his suspension pending investigation.

Therefore, the critical factor in this situation was not solely the act of drinking itself but rather the potential consequences of the doctor's drinking on the well-being of their patients and the associated risks linked to driving while impaired by alcohol.

If a referral is required, it is usually sensible for the practitioner–patient to self-refer to the regulator, advising them of the problem and confirming that they are under the care of a GP/psychiatrist/other addiction professional, that they have taken themselves out of the workplace to obtain treatment and have informed their occupational health physician and others as necessary. The regulator will consider the information and make its decision accordingly. It is best to be open and honest while at the same time ensuring that the practitioner–patient has access to appropriate guidance, treatment and support.

In deciding whether to refer to the regulator, seek advice and talk to colleagues within the team (if you have someone). It is also possible to get advice from the regulator by presenting an anonymised case history).

In the UK, the General Medical Council have several employer liaison advisors (ELA) who can offer advice (even anonymously), see:

- *https://www.gmc-uk.org/responsible-officer-hub/ros*

The role of the ELA is to:

- Establish good links with Responsible Officers and their teams to support exchanging information about underperforming doctors, improving patient safety and the quality of referrals.
- Share data about underperforming doctors, including regional trends.
- Help Responsible Officers and their teams understand GMC thresholds and procedures.
- To support the Responsible Officers and employers about revalidation.

GMC ELAs ensure that appropriate cases are referred to the GMC and support ROs/MDs to deal with appropriate cases at the local level rather than escalating to the GMC where not required.

The ELA can provide advice and guidance about GMC thresholds and act as a point of contact for any concerns or contact related to the GMC, see:

- https://nwpgmd.nhs.uk/sites/default/files/DiD_GMC.pdf

Practitioner Health has Memorandums of Understanding (MOU) with the healthcare regulators, including the GMC and GDC, which allows the service to treat some practitioner–patients without referral to the regulator unless the practitioner–patient fails to comply with the agreed treatment goals:

- *https://www.gmc-uk.org/about/how-we-work/who-we-work-with/our-memoranda-of-understanding*

- *https://www.gdc-uk.org/docs/default-source/who-we-work-with/gdc—php-mou.pdf?sfvrsn=db7d51c2_2*

DOCTORS WITH SUBSTANCE MISUSE AND REGULATORY INVOLVEMENT

Clinicians working with health professionals whose ability to practice is restricted by their regulator or by their employer have an important advocacy role to play. They should, therefore, make it their business to understand the relevant processes/procedures. Information can be obtained by visiting regulatory body websites, attending seminars and discussing the issues within a confidential team setting or a professional development and reflective practice group. This helps to demystify the process.

Practitioner–patients may feel too ashamed to ask for a written report for a hearing, and legal input is essential here. Treating clinicians should be aware of the power of the telephone call to the regulator or of a favourable report. It helps to validate the 'shared' nature of the ongoing work between the treating clinician and the practitioner–patient. A telephone call to the regulator to clarify a matter that has been worrying the practitioner–patient may help to relieve anxiety about a recent letter, document, or a forthcoming hearing.

The regulator is often the '*elephant in the room*' and looms large in the lives of regulated professionals, many of whom struggle with shame and humiliation. Some never recover. Resilient professionals, however, come to an acceptance of the situation. From despair at the outset and facing the loss of their career, relationships, houses and family, they begin to put the pieces of their lives back together. This does not happen overnight. Continuity of care is essential. This allows self-reflection and much-shared joy when they end the restricted practice, obtain the job they want, embark on new relationships, and generally regain their self-esteem and self-confidence. Some go on to help the next generation of practitioner–patients.

Regulatory bodies require the practitioner–patient to undergo regular blood or hair testing to confirm abstinence. This function is usually outsourced to a drug-testing company that will arrange to visit the practitioner–patient at home or in the workplace. Testing can be very stressful, even if the individual is '*clean*'.

Practitioner–patients may come to a session feeling very angry that they have been suspended because of what they perceive to have been a harsh report by their medical supervisor following a positive hair test. They may say they '*did not relapse*' but '*just used once or twice*'; it was a weekend, and there were no patient risks. Offer support, not judgment or criticism, and help the doctor regain their self-esteem despite potential negative consequences following their relapse. Stress that abstinence is a lifelong endeavour.

Treating professionals may find it challenging to agree on treatment goals – this can happen when the regulatory restrictions are not fully understood. Failure of treating professionals to consent does not help the practitioner–patient who remains ambivalent about their drug/alcohol problem and dismissive about treatment.

An open and honest therapeutic relationship between the addicted clinician and the professional(s) treating them is vital. This includes sharing information with loved ones, employers and others, if necessary. The treating clinician can be in several roles: therapist, counsellor, supporter, mentor and adviser. This partnership work aims to help the practitioner–patient become more self-aware and reflective. It will involve:

- Giving time and space to listen.

- Creating mutual respect and helping the practitioner–patient to maintain their dignity and self-esteem.

- It is creating and implementing an agreed care plan, which should include consideration of what will happen post-relapse.

- Providing support to understand, navigate and manage the regulatory process.

It is sensible for one clinician to take the lead on the case management, prescribing and network liaison fronts, arranging for additional help such as CBT, psychotherapy, or group work.

ABSTINENCE *VERSUS* SUBSTITUTE TREATMENT AND CONTROLLED DRINKING

Treatment services for doctors follow a largely abstinence-based approach, though there is no reason why, if necessary, opiate-addicted patients might be placed on long-term substitute medication. There are also some, albeit rarer, indications for controlled drinking rather than absence for alcohol-use disorder, depending on the level of drinking.[84]

The prescribing of psychotropic, substitute or anti-craving medication may be necessary to maintain recovery.

SUPPORTING RECOVERY

Peer support is central to recovery. The practitioner–patient is wise to attend mutual aid groups, and it may take months, even years, for them to engage fully in a 12-Step Fellowship or other groups such as the British Doctors & Dentists Group (BDDG). Those who affiliate tend to do well.

Addicted clinicians need wide-based support. As well as a specific treatment for their addiction and co-morbid mental health problems, they might need help and support to manage their relationship with their employers or supervisors. These doctors might be in debt, going through a divorce, trying to reconnect with children and family, mending broken relationships, finding a job, sitting exams, or coping with suspension, with the loss of everything that gave them a sense of worth. This is a lot to deal with.

They will need help to cope with the anxiety, anger, fury and despair, all of which are everyday experiences in the early days of recovery. These emotions might go on for some considerable time. Clinicians who do well ultimately come to terms with and accept the situation in which they are in. They also learn to navigate the complex web of treatment and monitoring requirements.

Evidence exists around engaging in '12-step approaches', which includes Alcoholics Anonymous or Narcotics Anonymous engagement. Attendance can be seen as more important than professionally directed treatments.

Three psychological variables influence the positive factors associated with the 12-step movement, these are[85]:

1. Shared belief

2. Group cohesiveness

3. Mutual identification

Research has also identified seven elements essential in a healthcare programme to prevent relapse including[86]:

1. A treatment plan

2. An assigned physician healthcare monitor

3. Abstinence

4. Analysis of body fluids

5. Attendance at mutual self-help meetings

6. A personal doctor

7. Advocacy

RELAPSE

A **relapse** is a return to substance use after a period of abstinence.

A relapse signifies that the individual still needs something to alleviate distress, usually because some critical personal issues have not yet been addressed. For a person with an opioid addiction, abstaining should also extend to abstaining from alcohol. Although outcomes for doctors are generally better than those of the general population, relapse still occurs, with potentially severe consequences including accidental overdose, harm to patients or families or suicide.

In a study of nearly 300 addicted doctors who had had treatment, 74 (25%) had at least one relapse. Most relapses occurred in the first year or two. Only 3% have their first relapse after five years. The state PHP health monitoring programme picked up most relapses.[87]

At Practitioner Health, doctors, if they do relapse, do so within weeks of ending treatment, '*just testing*' being a common motive for re-use. After the first six months post-treatment, the likelihood of abstinence by five years follow-up was nearly 80% for alcohol and 90% for drug misuse.[88]

Like other substance-dependent individuals, coexisting psychiatric morbidity ('*dual diagnosis*') is linked to a poor prognosis. A family history of addiction is also a bad prognostic factor. Researchers examined the follow-up of a group of health professionals who had completed a Physician Health Programme and went on to relapse. Those found to have been dishonest (not disclosing relapse, falsifying prescriptions), failure to engage in a 12-step programme and denial of the problem contributed to relapse. However, only 25% of physicians who had relapsed in the Arizona programme responded to their survey, meaning their numbers were small. There are dangers in applying these trends from a highly selected sample.[89]

There is no place for minimising the importance of relapse by calling it '*a bit of a slip*', and caution should be exercised in cases of poly-addiction that a doctor is using substances not included in their hair testing or not their primary original drug of abuse. These 'cross-addictions' and behaviours include gambling, sex, excessive spending and food. Compulsive behaviour around these activities can cause as much damage to the doctor's domestic and professional life as the original substance abuse.[16]

MUTUAL GROUPS SUPPORTING ADDICTION

The Sick Doctors Trust (SDT)

The **Sick Doctors Trust** (SDT) was established in 1996 by a group of doctors recovering from addictions concerned by the lack of adequate arrangements for helping others who found themselves in difficulty because of alcohol or drug use.

Through their work, they aim to:

- Both protect patients and offer hope to affected colleagues.
- Identify doctors suffering from the effects of addiction to alcohol and other drugs.
- Persuade affected doctors that they have an illness which can be treated successfully and to assist them in accessing such treatment.
- Assist doctors with the practical problems they may face in maintaining their livelihoods and supporting their families during treatment and recovery.
- Help to recover, doctors formulate a lifestyle conducive to uninterrupted continuing recovery.
- Assist, consult and cooperate with any agencies that share the objectives of SDT.

The British Doctors & Dentists Group (BDDG)

The **BDDG** are a group of doctors and dentists recovering from or wishing to recover from addiction and dependency on alcohol and other drugs. There are active groups in the UK and the Republic of Ireland. They share experiences and strengths and hope to understand their common problems and help and encourage other members and colleagues to recover from alcoholism and drug addiction. At each meeting, there is a free-flowing discussion on personal issues in recovery, some of which may be relevant to health professionals (e.g., fear, shame, guilt, stigma, problems with personal and professional relationships, involvement with the General Medical and General Dental Councils). Their meetings are not scientific discussions about alcoholism and drug addiction but focus on sharing their personal and professional journeys and difficulties and what has helped them recover.

They also have a support line for family members of addicted doctors and dentists.

The Dentists' Health Support Trust (DHST)

The **Dentists' Health Support Trust** (DHST) is a charity run by dentists for dentists. This charity can help dentists struggling with mental health and addiction issues across the four nations of the UK. The advice line is staffed 365 days a year. Callers will either speak with a fellow dentist or one of the national coordinators, who will offer confidential support and advice. In cases where formal mental health treatment or addiction interventions are needed, the staff at the Trust will help the dentist access these.

Other mutual support groups

Four prominent '**Anonymous**' groups are Alcoholics Anonymous, Narcotics Anonymous, Cocaine Anonymous and Gamblers Anonymous.

These groups provide mutual support for people with substance and process addictions. They follow a well-established 12-step programme. There are daily groups of varying sizes. Some of these groups are gender specific. How the group is run varies from group to group. They include discussion groups, noteworthy topics, and *main share groups* where an individual tells their story and gets feedback from others present. Individuals are encouraged to have a sponsor to support the group process. There are groups for family members, including Al-Anon Families and Adult Children of Alcoholics.

SMART Recovery is a science-based programme to help people manage their recovery from any addictive behaviour. This includes addictive behaviour with substances such as alcohol, nicotine or drugs or compulsive behaviours such as gambling, sex, eating, shopping, self-harming and so on. SMART stands for 'Self-Management and Recovery Training'. SMART began in 1994 in the United States. It is a four-point programme: building and maintaining motivation; coping with urges; managing thoughts, feelings and behaviours; and living a balanced life.

RETURN TO WORK

In the case of alcohol and drug dependence, remaining or returning to clinical duties is usually contingent upon abstinence from alcohol, illicit and over-the-counter drugs (unless prescribed or agreed) and evidence that co-morbid psychiatric and physical disorders are being treated/are in remission.

Returning to work after struggling with substance use and addiction can be a challenging and stressful experience, especially if there is a lack of support and monitoring. Individuals need a network of professionals to help them navigate this process and provide ongoing support as they recover. This can include supervising consultants, colleagues, clinical and medical directors, occupational health professionals and regulatory bodies. It can also be helpful for individuals to have access to mental health treatment and peer groups to cope with the stress and challenges of returning to work.

OUTCOME

Once addicted doctors are in treatment, they have excellent recoveries. Around 80% achieve abstinence, with a follow-up of about five years.[90] This is far higher than the general population, about 20%. Of those not at work, about 70% return to regular medical practice or training. A follow-up study of nearly 1,000 doctors attending North American PHs found that three-quarters maintained drug-free status; of those completing monitoring, 95% were licensed and working at five years follow-up.[81,88]

People with an addiction do not *'grow out of'* dependence, nor is the time spent in treatment a cure. Recovery is an ongoing process, not a neatly compartmentalised event, often requiring significant life changes. For some clinicians, the secrecy and shame of their addiction are so ingrained that they cling to the *status quo*, hoping that everyone and everything '*will just go away*'. It is tough to help clinicians who remain ambivalent about change and avoid therapeutic engagement. This group is often supported by the structured monitoring, testing and supervision provided by the fitness-to-practice procedures of their regulatory body. This group is at risk of relapse once restrictions are lifted. Failure to identify and treat mental health problems significantly affects recovery.

EXTRA RESOURCES AND SUPPORT SERVICES

1. *British Dentists and Doctors Group* http://www.bddg.org/

2. *Sick Doctors Trust* http://sick-doctors-trust.co.uk/

3. *Dentists' Health Support Trust* www.dentistshealthsupporttrust.org

4. *Alcoholics Anonymous* https://www.alcoholics-anonymous.org.uk/

5. *Narcotics Anonymous* http://ukna.org/

6. *Cocaine Anonymous* http://www.cauk.org.uk/index.asp

7. *Gamblers Anonymous* https://www.gamblersanonymous.org.uk/

8. *Sex Addicts Anonymous* http://saauk.info/en/

9. *SMART Recovery Groups* https://www.smartrecovery.org.uk/

MANAGEMENT OF BIPOLAR DISORDER

When reading this chapter, consider the following case, the risks involved and how they might be dealt with:

Morgan sat in his untidy office; his gaze fixated on the computer, his screen displaying patient notes. It had been a difficult day at the hospital, marked by his experiencing alternating moments of boundless energy and overwhelming despair. As a doctor with bipolar disorder, he navigated the challenging terrain of his mind while caring for the well-being of others.

His medical journey had been burdensome, shaped by periods of intense creativity, focus and drive during manic episodes, followed by debilitating bouts of depression that seemed to suffocate his soul. The highs and lows of his disorder had often mirrored the chaotic rhythm of his chosen profession.

Today had been a particularly challenging day. He had experienced a surge of energy, his lightning racing at lightning speed, as he effortlessly diagnosed complex cases and devised innovative treatment plans. But the euphoria had led to an abrupt descent into a cavern of melancholy, where each patient's pain resonated deeply within him, amplifying his inner turmoil.

He leaned back in his chair, feeling the weight of exhaustion settle upon his shoulders. The fluorescent lights above flickered, casting an eerie glow in the room. Jonathan's mind became a battleground, torn between the desire to escape the oppressive grip of his disorder and the responsibility to continue serving those in need.

He thought back to the early days of his career when he first received his diagnosis. The uncertainty and fear had been overwhelming, but he refused to let bipolar disorder define him. In those early days, he was terrified of being 'found out', constantly feeling that he was hiding a crime and that this was a sign of weakness to be unwell. After all, 'I am the doctor', he thought.

He took a deep breath, his hand reaching for the bottle of prescribed medication on his desk. It was a reminder of the delicate equilibrium he sought to maintain – a dance of medication, therapy and self-care. He knew adherence to his treatment plan was crucial for his well-being and the patients who depended on him.

Morgan is one of many doctors with bipolar disorder who can continue working in his chosen profession. He is engaged in treatment and follows the advice of his treating clinician. However, doctors, as mentioned earlier in this book, struggle to be treated compassionately and competently by their colleagues.

Morgan is a fictional case; Daksha, who has already been mentioned in this handbook, was not. Daksha had bipolar disorder. Through her medical school training, she had had many admissions, some of them compulsory, into a psychiatric hospital and was treated with electroconvulsive therapy. Despite the impact of these on her studies, she won several prestigious prizes. She married and continued her studies for the next eight years, and while taking medication, she never experienced a relapse. However, after discussing it with her psychiatrist, this long remission was disrupted when she stopped her medication to conceive and breastfeed her baby daughter. Three months later, she suffered an episode of postpartum psychosis, which led her to take the life of her three-month-old baby daughter and then her own. This happened the day before she was due to resume medication. During the previous month, she had been in touch with the community psychiatric nurse and psychiatrist due to poor sleep and depression. Still, she opted to manage without medication to continue breastfeeding.

Daksha had health professionals nominally in charge of her care. She had an NHS consultant psychiatrist, a general practitioner, an occupational health physician and a health visitor. But sadly, due to her medical status, she was treated differently from other patients with a similar severe condition. In a wish to protect her confidentiality and anonymity, her treating clinicians did not communicate with each other. Quite literally, she fell between the gaps of care.

That she was treated differently is not surprising, given what has already been discussed in this book. Even given the problems relating to stigma and shame which keep doctors away from services, many practical reasons prevent them from receiving the same care as their non-medical peers. Frequent changes of addresses due to training requirements reduce continuity of care. Colleagues misinterpret the need for confidentiality to mean not sharing information with those who might need to know (such as in Daksha's case, between health visitors, GPs and her treating psychiatrist). There is also often a belief that doctors, especially psychiatrists, know how to treat mental illness and should essentially manage themselves, with perhaps a light touch from external sources.

Kay McCall, a general practitioner with bipolar disorder, wrote about how she would have liked to have been treated by her colleagues in an article called 'An Insider's Guide to Depression'.[58]

Her article should be made compulsory reading for anyone caring for doctors. The reflection on depression by Katy McCall (McCall K. An insider's guide to depression. *BMJ*. 2001 Oct 27;323(7319):1011) is available for Open Access at: *https://www.ncbi.nlm.nih.gov/pmc/articles/PMC1121489/*.

Here are a few examples of the advice she gives:

> *Don't assume depressed doctors know that they're sick. The view is quite different from this side of the sanity divide. Chances are that we think we are only stressed by work and are distressed by our perceived inability to cope.*
>
> *People with depression don't have any sense of judgment or proportion. We desperately try to look as if we're in control, and often we don't know that our perceptions are false and our interpretations distorted.*
>
> *Don't be nervous about being empathetic. We won't clutch at you like drowning men. We want you only as a doctor. Make us feel like worthwhile people with a treatable illness.*
>
> *Feel free to ask us if we're suicidal. Suicidal thoughts for most of us have become everyday distress, and we're relieved to be able to talk about them.*
>
> *Give us hope. We need to be told unequivocally that we will get better.*
>
> *When you give us drugs, tell us about common side effects. If you don't do so and we get these side effects, our embryonic sense of hope is badly damaged.*
>
> *See us frequently at first.*
>
> *Please give us a reliable number we can call. This makes us feel that someone sees us as valuable.*

Doctors with mental illness must be managed as other patients, albeit with a focus on their professional and personal responsibilities. This means reviewing the diagnoses and ensuring they are on the appropriate treatment. A careful history and collateral information from family, friends and supervisors can be valuable in understanding the patient's experiences and in identifying any previous episodes of mania, hypomania, or depression. Misdiagnosis is common, as bipolar disorder can be mistaken for other conditions such as recurrent depression or personality disorder. It can also be challenging to identify hypomanic symptoms, as they may not always cause an impairment in functioning. Treating clinicians should assess the patient's ideas and thoughts to determine if they may be unrealistic or delusional; they must also be aware of the possibility of masking, where individuals may direct manic or hypomanic symptoms into increased work productivity.

It is essential to involve the general practitioner wherever possible, especially if the doctor needs a complex medication regime.

When doctors with BPAD receive the proper treatment, their mood improves, and they can return to work, with or without reasonable adjustments.

14

Presenteeism

Those supporting mentally ill doctors, whilst not occupational health clinicians, should know how and whether a doctor might return to work or need a period of sick leave from work.

Doctors have lower rates of sick leave than other employees. This might be related to their better health. However, there is also evidence that they have higher rates of what is termed '*presenteeism*', that is, attending work when unwell than others in similar stressful occupations.

Presenteeism can have several negative consequences for both employees and employers, including:

- Reduced productivity and quality of work
- Increased risk of errors and accidents
- The spread of illness to co-workers
- Decreased job satisfaction and morale
- Increased stress and burnout among employees

Employers and organisations often seek to address presenteeism by promoting a healthy work–life balance, providing access to support services, encouraging open communication about health and well-being, and creating a work environment that values employee well-being and engagement over mere physical presence. Addressing presenteeism can improve employee health, satisfaction and overall workplace productivity.

There are reasons why doctors work when unwell. The most common is guilt at leaving colleagues under-resourced if they were absent. But there are other reasons. Paradoxically, the job itself – even given its high demand, might be less stressful than other jobs, which might be more mundane. This links to the **Aronsson and Gustafsson conceptual model** (also known as the **demand-control model**),[91]

DOI: 10.1201/9781003391500-14

which sets out to explain the relationship between work-related stressors and health outcomes.

The model proposes that work-related stress results from two key factors: Job demands and job control. Job demands refer to the workload and pressure placed on an employee, while job control refers to an employee's autonomy and decision-making power. The model suggests that employees with high job demands and low job control are at the most significant risk for experiencing stress-related health problems, such as cardiovascular disease and mental health issues. This is because these individuals may feel overwhelmed and unable to cope with the demands placed on them. Conversely, employees with high job demands and job control may experience less stress because they have more control over their work and can make decisions to manage their workload. Doctors tend to have high demands and high control of their position, which might influence their decision to work when unwell.

However, there are also potential negative consequences of presenteeism among doctors. If a doctor is unwell or experiencing symptoms of illness, they may be less effective in their role and could compromise patient safety. Additionally, if a doctor is contagious and continues to work, they could put their patients and colleagues at risk of infection.

Furthermore, if presenteeism is driven by a culture that values long work hours and pressures doctors to work even when they are not feeling well, it can contribute to burnout and decreased job satisfaction. This, in turn, can negatively impact patient care and outcomes.

Assessing whether a doctor should take sick leave is up to the treating clinician, working with their patient. It is often a good idea to have a respite if only to re-calibrate one's mental health, catch up on sleep and have time to reflect on what might help reduce the further risk of mental illness.

15

Returning to work

Doctors are motivated to resume work and often pressure their treating clinician (and employer) to allow them to do so even when it might not be appropriate due to ongoing health problems. Of course, one does not need to be 100% fit to return to work – but there is a balance between returning too early, risking performing sub-optimally (possibly leading to complaints) and ensuring they are allowed back into the workplace and engaging in their everyday activities. When back at work, doctors might want to rush full steam ahead and work to total capacity even though it would be better to ease themselves back gradually. These doctors might engage in behaviours that include taking extra shifts, handling challenging patients and seeking ways to demonstrate to the team that they are making up for lost time. Occupational health can help prepare return-to-work plans to temper the doctor's enthusiasm to do too much too soon.

Regular reviews during sick leave help ensure the practitioner–patient receives the support they need and makes progress. These reviews can identify barriers or concerns that may impact the return-to-work process and allow adjustments to be made to the plan as needed.

When seeing practitioner–patients who are thinking about a return to work, it is essential to ask and discuss the following:

1. **Presenting illness/Cause for time off and the response to treatment:** For example, the various reasons which led to the illness and the need to take time away from work.
2. **Workplace triggers:** Contributing to needing time off. This could include issues related to partnerships, team difficulties, mergers, rota gaps or other workplace stressors.
3. **Roles and responsibilities:** This will help identify areas where adjustments may be needed to support a return to work.
4. **Liaison with health professionals:** It might be helpful to gather information from occupational health or other health professionals. This will help

140 DOI: 10.1201/9781003391500-15

ensure the return-to-work plan considers any medical restrictions or recommendations.

5. **Previous experience:** It is helpful to learn from any previous experiences the practitioner–patient may have had with returning to work. This information can help anticipate any potential difficulties and plan accordingly.

6. **Previous episodes of sickness and how they were managed:** This information will help identify recurring patterns or issues that must be addressed.

7. **Phased return:** A phased return is often the most effective way to support a practitioner–patient's return to work. This involves gradually increasing their workload over weeks or months, with additional duties or roles added slowly. Ideally, this must be done with the patient's occupational health practitioner and employer.

Creating a successful return-to-work plan requires understanding the practitioner-patient's medical condition, workplace environment and job responsibilities. Considering these factors and working closely with other health professionals (with consent), a plan can be devised to support the practitioner–patient's triumphant return to work.

Always remember that there needs to be a balance between allowing sufficient time for recovery and avoiding prolonged periods of absence that can result in reduced confidence and increased worry.

Ultimately, the goal should be to support the practitioner–patient in returning to work at a safe, realistic and sustainable pace while also considering the workplaces and colleagues' needs.

TIMING OF RETURN TO WORK

Returning too soon may decrease the chance of success if the unwell health professional has yet to recover sufficiently. Yet, simultaneously, it is essential to minimise absences and have the least time off work that is necessary. Taking long periods from work is associated with reduced confidence in their ability to manage their role and can lead to excess rumination and worry whilst off sick. There is, therefore, a delicate balance between having time off sick and returning to work. Once at work, the doctor must work at full competence. A depressed doctor who still finds it hard to focus on their work is unsafe and, as such, should not be at work.

PLANNING RETURN TO WORK

Returning to work after a period of sick leave due to mental illness can be challenging, but with proper planning and support, it is possible to have a successful transition. It is common for the patient to experience increased anxiety once the decision has been made to agree on a return-to-work date. This anticipatory anxiety follows a typical curve, increasing in the days preceding the return and then easing once back in the workplace and getting on with daily tasks. Rehearsing how to answer questions from colleagues about reasons for absence (e.g., on return after inpatient detoxification from alcohol or drugs) is also helpful.

There is often a tendency to over-share, why one has not been working. It is helpful to rehearse what to say before returning to work, especially if away for a prolonged period.

The aim is for the practitioner–patient to share enough information to have the appropriate support on return to work and to maintain the trust of their close colleagues whilst reserving the right to privacy concerning their clinical details.

FITNESS TO WORK RELATED TO PERFORMANCE ISSUES

Under certain circumstances, mental or physical health problems, there might need to be a decision to stop working altogether. For example, suppose a practitioner-patient had a neurological condition affecting the manual dexterity required for their role (such as to conduct surgery). In that case, they may consider applying for retirement on medical grounds as they could not continue to perform their function. A severe and enduring mental health problem requires special consideration and adaptions in the workplace.

16

The role of occupational health

Occupational health practitioners can provide valuable support and guidance for doctors who want to return to work after sickness, injury, or other health-related absence. They are experts in the interface between work and health. These practitioners can assess the individual's health and work-related needs and recommend any necessary adjustments to support their return to work and promote their ongoing health and well-being.[92]

Below are some critical aspects of the role of occupational health in supporting doctors returning to work:

1. **Assessment and evaluation:** Occupational health professionals can assess the doctor's health condition to determine their readiness to return to work. This assessment involves reviewing medical records, conducting interviews and possibly consulting with other clinicians caring for the doctor.

2. **Treatment and rehabilitation planning:** Working out what short and medium-term interventions can be provided to aid recovery.

3. **Return-to-Work planning:** Occupational health specialists can assist in creating a structured and gradual return-to-work plan. This plan considers the doctor's needs, limitations and abilities, ensuring a smooth transition to their professional responsibilities.

4. **Workplace accommodations:** In some cases, reasonable accommodations may be necessary to support the doctor's health. Occupational health professionals can work with the doctor's employer to identify and implement reasonable accommodations, such as modified work hours or reduced patient loads.

5. **Monitoring and support:** Occupational health monitors the doctor's progress after their return to work. Regular check-ins and ongoing support are essential to ensure they cope well and can adjust if needed.

6. **Education and training:** Occupational health may provide education and training to colleagues and staff to promote a supportive and stigma-free work environment. This can help reduce potential biases or misunderstandings related to mental health conditions.

7. **Confidentiality and privacy:** Ensuring the confidentiality and privacy of the doctor's medical information is critical. Occupational health professionals adhere to strict ethical and legal standards to protect the doctor's health information.

8. **Compliance with regulations:** Occupational health experts ensure that relevant workplace and medical regulations are followed, including those related to disability accommodations, medical leave and medical certification.

Many doctors are worried about the confidentiality of an occupational health assessment and advice. They fear that being so closely linked to their employment, their employer might be given their personal information. This is not the case. If concerned, the easiest way to resolve these anxieties is for the patient to discuss them with their doctor and ask for a copy of the OH confidentiality policy before the OH consultation.

If an individual struggles at work for any reason, including health-related issues, engaging with occupational health practitioners to explore what support and adjustments can be implemented to help manage their health and well-being is important. This can include flexible working arrangements, adjustments to their work environment or duties, or additional support from their employer or colleagues.

When considering returning to work, it might be helpful for the treating practitioners to advise their patients to consider some of the issues listed below:

1. **Prioritise well-being:** Ensure you have sought appropriate treatment, therapy and support during your time off.

2. **Be open when communicating with your employer:** Discuss your absence, recovery progress and any accommodations or adjustments you may need upon returning to work.

3. **Plan a gradual return to work:** Consider a phased or gradual return, depending on your illness' severity and circumstances. This approach allows you to gradually increase your workload and responsibilities, giving you time to readjust and manage potential challenges.

4. **Collaborate with your healthcare provider:** Work closely with your healthcare provider, therapist, or psychiatrist to develop a plan for your return to work. They can provide recommendations, write a letter outlining your capabilities and limitations and suggest any necessary accommodations to support your successful transition into your role.

5. **Seek workplace adjustments if needed:** If you require workplace adjustments, such as reduced hours, modified duties, or a flexible schedule, discuss these with your employer.

6. **Develop coping strategies:** Identify coping strategies that work for you to manage stress and maintain your well-being. This may include setting

boundaries, practising self-care during breaks, taking time off when needed and seeking support from colleagues, friends, or mental health professionals when necessary.

7. **Connect with supportive colleagues:** Establishing a support network within your workplace is crucial. Reach out to trusted colleagues or mentors who can provide guidance and support as you transition back to work. Consider joining support groups or employee assistance programmes if available.

8. **Monitor your workload:** Be mindful of your workload and avoid taking on excessive responsibilities immediately upon your return. Communicate your capacity to your supervisor or team members, and gradually increase your workload as you feel comfortable and capable.

9. **Maintain a work-life balance:** A healthy work–life balance prevents burnout and promotes well-being. Set boundaries, establish self-care routines and engage in activities outside of work that bring you joy and relaxation.

10. **Monitor your progress:** Keep track of your progress as you return to work. Regularly assess how you're feeling, both physically and mentally.

Everyone's journey is unique, and being patient and kind to yourself during this transition is essential. With the proper support and self-care, one can successfully resume work as a doctor while prioritising one's mental health.

17

Talking therapies

Talking therapies are the backbone of treatment for anyone with psychological or mental health issues. Psychotherapy is the umbrella term for a range of treatment modalities. It is not limited to talking therapies as they can employ other forms of expression such as art, music and dance.

These therapies address many emotional, psychological and mental health issues. Talking therapies help people better understand and manage their thoughts, feelings and behaviours, improving their mental well-being and coping skills.

PSYCHODYNAMIC PSYCHOTHERAPY

Psychodynamic therapy is based on the theory and practice of psychoanalysis, founded by Sigmund Freud in the late nineteenth century and then developed over the years by others. From its routes in treating so-called *hysterics*, it is now applied to various types of mental distress. It has good evidence as a treatment for depression, anxiety, panic disorders and personality disorders. Moreover, evidence suggests that the therapeutic gains seen in psychodynamic psychotherapy are maintained longer and continue to improve after therapy.

Psychodynamic psychotherapy takes a developmental approach. Current problems can often be traced to the environment we grew up in, particularly our relationships with caregivers. It is based on the theory that large parts of our mind are inaccessible to our conscious thought processes. This part of the mind, the unconscious, is where our primitive drives function, our uncomfortable memories are repressed, and our unpalatable wishes are held. The unconscious has an enormous influence on our behaviour in the present, and it is accessed in psychodynamic psychotherapy through the techniques of free association, dream work and interpretation. There is a focus on the patient's transference and the therapist's countertransference. Transference involves the patient unconsciously displacing onto the therapist echoes of their past meaningful relationships; countertransference is the reaction that may be evoked in the therapist. Both are essential tools within psychodynamic psychotherapy for understanding the unconscious processes at work.

DOI: 10.1201/9781003391500-17

Psychodynamic psychotherapy is a gradual, long-term, and often challenging process and is helpful for patients wishing to gain a deeper understanding of themselves and how they relate to others. It looks more at underlying psychological and unconscious issues and is not primarily focused on symptom relief.

It takes place at a set time, in a set location for 45–50 minutes each week, and sometimes several times a week. This can be for many years.

COGNITIVE BEHAVIOURAL THERAPY (CBT)

Cognitive behavioural therapy (CBT) was developed from the work of psychologist Albert Ellis and psychiatrist Aaron Beck. Based on behavioural and cognitive psychology, CBT has emerged as the dominant psychotherapy available within the NHS in recent years. It is structured, collaborative, usually brief, and focuses primarily on the present, using a model that links conscious thoughts to feelings and behaviours. The model explains to patients how challenging or unpleasant feelings and behaviours are often based on irrational thoughts, which are then reinforced by subsequent emotional and behavioural responses.

There is a focus on agenda, goal setting and homework between sessions. The therapist and patient develop a shared formulation of the patient's problem. This formulation aims to uncover the patient's core beliefs towards themselves and others, usually based on early experiences and their 'rules for living', which govern how these beliefs are applied. Using these beliefs, rules and exploration of automatic thoughts, the therapist aims to help the patient unlearn these pathological cognitions. They do this using testing, weighing lists of pros and cons through experiments and other direct interventions.

CBT has a well-established evidence base for treating depression, generalised anxiety, phobias, obsessional-compulsive disorder and post-traumatic stress disorder. However, as with most psychotherapies, it relies heavily on patients' insight, motivation and ability to think psychologically about their problems.

COUNSELLING

Counselling is a supportive process involving a counsellor and patient. It is generally non-directive and often works within the 'core conditions' as Carl Rogers defined in the person-centred approach's development. These are empathy, congruence and unconditional positive regard.

It can be a brief intervention or over a longer time. It shows good evidence for common mental health problems such as depression and anxiety and significant life changes such as grief, leaving home or divorce. Generally, it is a less challenging approach but still requires the patient to be motivated to attend and disclose their distress.

NOVEL STRUCTURED THERAPIES

Mentalisation-based therapy (MBT)

Developed by the psychoanalytic psychotherapists Anthony Bateman and Peter Fonagy and drawing on clinical experience combined with a solid evidence base, **mentalisation-based therapy** (MBT) is a manualised, structured, long-term psychotherapy. It was developed specifically for treating personality disorders and is now used for various conditions. It is based on the formulation of personality disorder as a disorder of attachment and social cognition, with a resultant deficit in mentalising, particularly when exposed to attachment-related stress. Mentalising is a new term for an ancient concept – the uniquely human capacity to understand and reflect on our mental states and the ability to see things from another perspective.

Under stress, all human beings go into what is termed 'non-mentalising modes', losing the ability to think reflectively when anxious, afraid, angry, in love, *etc.* Non-mentalising is demonstrated by a range of thinking patterns, such as an excessive certainty of thought, a heavy focus on external factors for problems (blaming/fault finding), a focus on labels, and a preoccupation with rules and denial. In certain individuals, non-mentalising modes happen more frequently or to a greater degree than in others and have a subsequent impact on functioning, often leading to self-destructive behaviours. MBT aims to encourage mentalising in the individual through various psychotherapeutic techniques. The therapist adopts a 'non-knowing stance', encouraging curiosity and collaboration throughout treatment. The therapist is very active in sessions – although they do not give advice, they aim to model mentalising. It is based on the present, focusing on current relational difficulties, although informed by a formulation based on early attachment patterns. Sessions last 60 minutes, and individuals often receive one-on-one and group sessions for up to 18 months.

Dialectical behavioural therapy

Dialectical behavioural therapy (DBT) was developed in the 1980s by American psychologist Marsha Linehan, specifically for treating severe personality disorders. CBT had traditionally failed to treat these patients, so the techniques were adjusted to include mindfulness practices more commonly found in Buddhism. There is an emphasis on the therapist as an ally rather than an adversary and a strong focus on acquiring skills. Participants receive both individual and group therapy every week. There are four 'modules', so in addition to mindfulness meditation, participants work on interpersonal effectiveness, distress tolerance and emotional self-regulation.

GROUP THERAPY

Group therapy covers any psychotherapy delivered to more than one individual simultaneously, though if only one other person, it is referred to as 'couples therapy'.

Group therapy can occur in groups of any size, though it usually involves at least six individuals but can be as large as many hundreds (called a 'large group').

As John Dunne wrote in the sixteenth century, '*No man is an island, entire of itself*', meaning that humans are drawn towards one another; we are social animals and form groups. It is generally accepted that membership in any group enhances human development and decision-making. Group therapy builds on this wisdom and attempts to harness individuals' power to benefit all members collectively.

The first groups to treat illness emerged in the early twentieth century, and the term 'Group Therapy' was coined in 1920 by Jacob Moreno. Moreno studied medicine, psychoanalysis and social networks during his life and was keenly interested in improvisational theatre. He combined all these in his work on psychodrama and group psychotherapy. The psychiatrist S. H. Foulkes, a German-born Jewish émigré who came to the UK in the early 1930s, began running psychotherapy groups for soldiers with trauma returning from the Second World War. After the war, he and others following him ran groups for NHS patients with 'neurotic' conditions (depression, marital problems, specific phobias) and developed group analysis/therapy discipline.

Group therapy focuses on the relationship between the individual and the rest of the group and brings in issues from the individual's community, family and social network. Membership typically involves patients drawn from different socio-cultural, age and gender communities and other presenting problems – so-called *heterogeneous groups*. The art of creating a therapeutic group culture is, in part, finding, exploring and articulating differences without losing the essential connections that keep members together and allow each to recognise that they are together, all social objects, part of a social world, seeking a group. However, for some individuals or those with some conditions (for example, eating disorders), groups with more similarities than differences help improve group cohesion. The premise is that the greater the shared foundations, the more this is possible, and the better the therapeutic impact.

Groups should be integral to the treatment offered to doctors. Perhaps more than any other patient group, doctors with mental illness fear disclosing their condition. Single-professional groups help overcome barriers and enable the individual to attach to the group and, as such, take on the patient role. Practitioner Health has been offering groups to doctors as part of their treatment.[81] These are a variety of different groups. Mixed and single gender, groups for trainees, senior (consultants and GPs), same and mixed speciality, specific problem (drug and alcohol, exam failure) and groups for suspended doctors. PH has also run a group for those bereaved following the death through the suicide of a health professional.[93] The groups vary in duration (time-limited and open-ended) and membership (closed, slowly open, honest). All use a mixture of psychotherapeutic and reflective practice techniques adapted to meet the needs of this patient population.

Descriptions of some of these groups are provided later in this handbook.

The American psychiatrist Irvin Yalom highlighted the following curative factors present in groups:[94]

- Imparting information
- Cohesion
- Instillation of hope
- Universality
- Altruism
- Socialising
- Imitative behaviour
- Interpersonal learning

A **Schwartz Round** is a type of structured forum or discussion used in healthcare settings to provide a space for healthcare professionals to share their thoughts and feelings openly and safely about the emotional and social challenges they encounter in their work, particularly in patient care. These rounds are named after Dr. Robert Schwartz, who initiated them.

The primary purpose of a Schwartz Round is to facilitate open and honest conversations about the emotional aspects of healthcare, allowing staff to discuss their experiences, dilemmas and personal responses to patient care. It is a form of peer support and reflection that helps healthcare professionals better understand and cope with their work's emotional and moral dimensions.

Schwartz Rounds are typically structured discussions led by a facilitator, often a team leader or healthcare professional, where participants can share their experiences, thoughts and feelings without judgement or needing solutions. The focus is on the emotional impact of the work and the human aspects of caregiving. These rounds can help healthcare teams build empathy, reduce feelings of isolation and improve their overall well-being, making them more effective and resilient.

Schwartz Rounds have gained popularity in healthcare organisations as a way to address the emotional toll of the profession and promote emotional well-being and support among healthcare staff.

A **Balint Group** is a specific type of group therapy or discussion group commonly used in medical and healthcare settings. It is designed to help healthcare professionals, particularly doctors and other clinicians, explore and reflect upon their relationships with patients. Balint Groups are named after the Hungarian psychoanalyst Michael Balint and his wife, Enid, who developed this approach in the 1950s.

The primary focus of a Balint Group is on the doctor–patient relationship and the emotional and interpersonal dynamics that come into play during clinical interactions. These groups typically consist of healthcare professionals who meet regularly to discuss patient cases and the associated feelings, thoughts and challenges that arise in their work.

Critical features of Balint Groups include the following:

1. **Case presentation:** In a Balint Group session, one member (usually a healthcare professional) presents a patient case, including the medical history and their own experiences and feelings related to the case.

2. **Reflective discussion:** The group engages in a structured, reflective discussion of the case. The discussion often includes exploring the healthcare professional's feelings, countertransference (emotional reactions to the patient) and the dynamics of the doctor–patient relationship.

3. **Non-Judgmental support:** Balint Groups provide a safe and confidential space for members to express their thoughts and emotions without fear of judgement. This allows participants to gain insight into their emotional responses and the impact of those responses on patient care.

4. **Learning and growth:** Balint Groups aim to help healthcare professionals better understand themselves and their patient interactions. This, in turn, can lead to improved communication, empathy and patient care.

Balint Groups enhance self-awareness, improve the doctor–patient relationship and reduce burnout among healthcare professionals. They offer a structured and supportive environment for clinicians to share their experiences, gain insight into their emotional responses and ultimately provide more effective and compassionate patient care.

18

Reflections

FROM A COGNITIVE BEHAVIOURAL THERAPIST (CBT) WORKING AT PH

Simon Lyne

In my experience of treating doctors and dentists, cognitive behavioural therapy (CBT) works best when it is flexible and tailored to the individual. In practice, this means creating a personalised formulation following assessment, which informs the course of therapy alongside what the patient brings to each session. Traditional CBT usually follows rigid protocols, but if a patient suffers a bereavement or a relationship breakdown midway through treatment for social anxiety, for example, this may change the direction and focus of that and potentially subsequent sessions.

Therapeutic work often benefits from weekly sessions, at least to start with. However, due to new technology, patients' erratic work lives and competing demands of personal life, it is helpful to discuss flexibility and ensure motivation and out-of-session tasks are utilised.

Doctors and dentists at Practitioner Health are usually high-functioning, intelligent individuals. This makes psychological work somewhat straightforward but comes with its own set of challenges.

Anxiety

Fear is part of the human experience and the natural response to anticipated danger. Physical and cognitive changes occur to protect us, which is a helpful survival mechanism. Feeling anxious is much like the feeling of fear but without the presence of actual danger.

The cognitive model of anxiety suggests that anxiety results from overestimating the threat and the danger's perceived consequences. It also indicates that we tend to underestimate our ability to cope and the resources available to help us when anxious.

DOI: 10.1201/9781003391500-18

Learning to quieten our sympathetic nervous system response and stimulate the parasympathetic is essential to manage anxiety. One evidence-based way to do this quickly and effectively is through slow, controlled breathing.

We must learn to appraise threats realistically, build and reinforce coping mechanisms, and face and deal with threats constructively rather than avoid them.

Worry and catastrophic thinking are generally reported when patients are experiencing anxiety. There are various ways to interrupt this cycle: By first being aware of it, reminding ourselves we are engaging with stories in our head (which the body responds to with the physiological aspects of anxiety), reminding ourselves how we can cope, and thinking of alternative narratives that might also be possible. Usually, people recognise worry as unhelpful and can think of adaptive problem-solving strategies for real issues. These can be dealt with in the real world, gently shifting attention away from fruitless extended thinking.

Depression

Cognitive therapy aims to help patients identify and reframe their negative, often self-critical and blaming thoughts and thought patterns. The behavioural side of things allows patients to re-engage in their lives meaningfully, connected with what we find valuable at our core. Depressed patients will usually withdraw and isolate themselves, negating any opportunity for positive interactions.

Often, we need to delve a little deeper to find out if there are any underlying negative core beliefs (usually stemming from early experiences). We can then work to develop more helpful core ideas and ways of thinking about the self, others, the world, and the future that can then be recognised and reinforced in everyday life through behaviour.

Patients might also find themselves ruminating on the past or asking themselves endless soul-searching questions about why they are feeling this way and what it means for how they see themselves (generally negative). Like worry, it takes time and practice to non-judgementally and compassionately move away from this type of perseverative thinking, which has been shown to exacerbate and prolong depression.

Perfectionism

As discussed earlier in this book, many doctors and dentists will identify as perfectionists, and there may be an erroneous belief that this is helpful. Unfortunately, striving for perfection (often at a high personal cost) is ultimately self-defeating since perfection is impossible. The perfectionist is continually stressed, anxious and usually disappointed with themselves. Perfectionists judge their self-worth primarily on achieving unrelenting high standards; it can be seen as an unhealthy striving for external validation rather than a healthy internal drive for excellence. Sometimes, perfectionists may not be able to start a project because their intense fear of not being able to do a 'perfect' job prevents them from beginning it. They may also need help finishing things for the same reason. Perfectionism is, therefore, closely linked with low self-esteem.

Self-esteem

Self-esteem has long been thought to be essential for feeling good about ourselves. In CBT, people are often encouraged to engage in things that give them a sense of pleasure and achievement, which invariably helps people feel better about themselves and their lives. Self-acceptance, however, is also a vital ingredient and arguably more important. Self-esteem is often conditional in that we can only feel good when things are going well when we are doing things well or judge ourselves to be doing better than others. This is clear in perfectionism, where people tell themselves they can only feel good if they achieve their unrelenting high standards. Perfectionists will have many negative thoughts about themselves and their abilities when they don't. Self-acceptance understands that we are imperfect human beings, acting imperfectly. Self-acceptance involves incorporating the good points and the bad, the strengths and the weaknesses, the assets and the liabilities, etc. Self-acceptance is not conditional and is there when we fail, are rejected or fall flat on our faces. These two create a powerhouse alongside self-compassion (being with our pain and wanting to do something positive to help ourselves). It is a cliché, but finding a way to be an excellent friend to yourself is one of the most valuable and protective things we can do.

Mindfulness

Mindfulness and mindful meditation are increasingly recognised as powerful tools in combating various human problems. Mindfulness uses the senses to attend to the experience of the present moment in a non-judgemental and purposeful manner. It is an antidote to being an 'automatic pilot', grounding us in the here and now and interrupting automatic and unhelpful ways of thinking and responding. When we are in 'experiencing mode', we also cannot worry about the future or fretting about the past.

There are many excellent smartphone apps that will guide the listener through mindful meditation. With mindful meditation, we will sit with what is happening in our bodies and minds and focus on breathing. We are also taught to detach from thoughts and recognise them for what they are – ideas and nothing more. Depending on the app, valuable insights into various things, such as loving-kindness or gratitude, may also be discussed. Like everything else, it takes time, patience, and regular practice to learn the concepts, but the benefits, such as increased self-awareness, less stress and a quieter mind, can be profound. Many patients will report they struggle with mindful meditation as they believe they're not 'doing it right', but our minds wander naturally – we need to notice that (without judgement) and gently bring it back.

There is valuable information on the 'Mindful' website *https://www.mindful.org.*

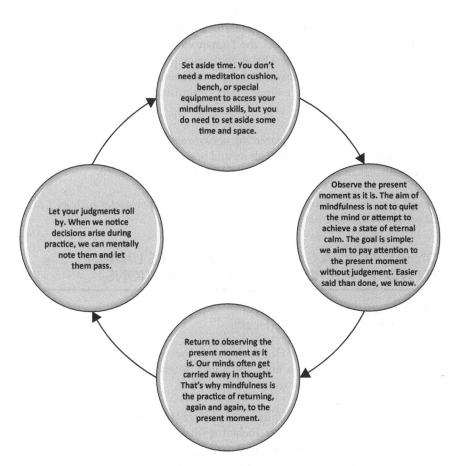

Figure 18.1 Approach to supporting the mentally ill doctor.

Doctors who treat doctors need to create a therapeutic frame. It is the responsibility of the treating doctor to keep up boundaries of this frame as, unconsciously or consciously, the patient will tend to want to move towards a more intimate, less professional discourse. It is also naturally tempting for treating doctors to go with this move. This may be as much to themselves and reduce anxiety as treating doctors are more comfortable seeing sick doctors as 'doctors' and not patients.

Maintaining boundaries is not just about confidentiality and statutory obligations. It is about retaining the parameters in which the consultation is taking place. Setting appointment times and limits, agreed methods of contact that are not crossed, use of professional titles, limited self-disclosure, etc., are all tools used within therapeutic settings to maintain boundaries vigilantly. Again, this is to provide containment through professionalism and avoid the 'slippery slope' of boundary violations.

In the patient's position, there can be a retreat into defensive intellectualisation, into the medical knowledge and language they are well versed in, to distract from the emotional pain involved. This intellectualisation can seduce the treating doctor and, in doing so, can neglect the human vulnerability of the practitioner–patient. Therefore, the language between the practitioner–patient and the treating doctor is essential in ensuring honest communication. For example, that light, mature humour hasn't slipped into minimising, avoiding, or dismissing the scale of a problem.

As with intellectualisation, the treating doctor can be pulled into the more flexible position of a friend who goes above and beyond or out of their way for a colleague rather than a trusted professional who maintains distance.

Unwell doctors can distract themselves with structural obstacles such as '*I can't take time off*'; '*confidentiality won't be maintained*'.

ON RUNNING A GROUP FOR DOCTORS UNABLE TO WORK DUE TO REGULATORY SANCTIONS

Sheila Jones
Psychotherapist, Practitioner Health

One aspect of Practitioners Health's work is the 'Suspended Doctors Group', which meets monthly for an hour and a half. Attendance at these meetings is optional, but doctors often attend to seek support.

During the group sessions, doctors are encouraged to share their stories and provide updates on their experiences, including what has or hasn't worked for them. The group aims to understand the underlying thoughts and emotions behind everyone's situation, explore strategies for managing distress and reflect on how they arrived at their present circumstances.

When doctors are suspended from practice, they commonly experience a shift in emotions from initial shame to hopelessness, helplessness and depression. The realisation of their suspension and its consequences can be overwhelming. They may direct their anger towards the General Medical Council (GMC), perceiving them as responsible for their predicament. However, this anger can distract them from examining their role in the events leading to their suspension. This can result in a deepening sense of despair, heightened depressed feelings, anger, frustration and growing resentment. The doctor may feel attacked and penalised by the suspension process.

The reasons for doctors' suspensions often involve drug and alcohol misuse, often fuelled by depression. Some doctors' pleas for help may have been ignored by colleagues or authorities with jurisdiction over them. Others may have concealed their deteriorating health behind increased substance abuse.

The majority of the Suspended Doctors Group consists of doctors from African/Caribbean, Asian or other overseas backgrounds, many of whom received their medical training abroad. Fewer doctors are from White British or European locations, and when they do join, they tend not to stay long, often citing personal reasons for their departure. This prevalence of overseas-trained doctors and those from ethnic minorities exacerbates perceptions of racism within the medical profession. Some doctors may feel scapegoated, betrayed, subjected to double standards or victims of injustice. Feeling ostracised by their colleagues intensifies their sense of persecution, and they may perceive the system as engaging in psychological games. The doctor, unable to comprehend the reasons behind the allegations they face, may suspect that their race or ethnicity is a contributing factor.

Women comprise a small proportion of the group, usually only one or two individuals at any time.

The group also occasionally invites external speakers to address various topics, such as practical advice on seeking legal assistance, preparing for hearings, accessing clinical attachments and coping with similar situations. These talks allow doctors to consider their current situation, long-term goals of returning to work and alternative career prospects.

A prevalent concern in the group is whether they can still refer to themselves as 'a doctor', particularly after being erased from the medical register. Other practical issues arise, including the absence of a workplace to go to, a gradual reduction and eventual loss of income, and a loss of contact with colleagues. Suspended doctors report experiencing avoidance from colleagues, who view them as a 'bad egg'. In some cases, senior staff forbid colleagues from interacting with the suspended doctor, reinforcing a sense of being unwanted.

Based on my experience working with suspended doctors, they tend to suffer from various mental health issues because of their suspension. These issues range from denial, shame, anger and resentment to guilt, depression and suicidal feelings. They feel a profound sense of injustice, believing the system has mistreated them. Being aware of colleagues who have gone undetected or unpunished for similar transgressions, the doctor facing suspension feels singled out and uncertain about their future. They perceive the system as punishing them for what they initially consider minor infractions or issues that could be explained without retribution. Some doctors may express their emotions through tears, while others may internalise negative feelings, leading to depression. In extreme cases, some doctors contemplate or carry out suicidal actions.

For suspended doctors to make progress, they must confront their involvement in the incidents leading to their suspension. Persistent denial hampers insight development, typically frowned upon during GMC/GDC hearings. Once a doctor has adjusted to the shock of their suspension, they must adapt to their new circumstances. This adjustment can be challenging due to the enduring negative emotions they experience, particularly related to shame and the loss of their professional identity. The role of being a doctor holds great significance for them, and when suspension, undertakings or erasure occurs, the sense of identity loss leaves the doctor adrift. These factors have led some doctors to take their own lives, causing devastating consequences for their loved ones and raising significant questions for the medical profession.

Finding employment while suspended poses a challenge for many doctors since their qualifications often make them appear overqualified for other positions. They may need clarification about why they are out of work or not seeking employment in their field. Suspended doctors can apply for any job except clinical work, which involves being 'a doctor'. It is essential that they engage in meaningful activities to fill their time, but not at the expense of avoiding painful feelings, which can perpetuate negative behavioural patterns. Voluntary work is one option available to suspended doctors. Financial constraints may require them to apply for state benefits, which can be daunting and emotionally taxing.

ON RUNNING REFLECTIVE GROUPS FOR DOCTORS

Clare Gerada
Medical Director, Practitioner Health

Bringing together eight or so busy people into a therapy group is complex and sometimes akin to the proverbial herding sheep. No sooner had all members attending a group than the following week, only three or four would. Group therapy requires regular attendance by its group members. Yet, this is rarely the case for groups made up of doctors. Early dropouts due to unforeseen problems, life events, illnesses and unexpected incidents can interfere with regular attendance. Factor into this, as far as doctors are concerned, irregular shift patterns of working (often changing with little notice), running late due to patient needs (patient's illnesses do not neatly fall into fixed time patterns), and the inevitability of having to cover absent colleagues and attendance can become erratic. This makes creating continuity difficult and, with it, creating trust difficult. Attendance was better for junior and senior doctors; women attended more regularly than male doctors. Infrequent attendance became part of the group dialogue and an attempt to understand this in the context of doctors' unconscious (rather than practical lives). For example:

Fatima challenged Allan on his lateness. He was always 5–10 minutes, citing excuses such as 'traffic, work' pressures. She told the group his lateness brought up memories of her father, who was unreliable in the family home and his abuse of her mother. She challenged Allan, saying it was also his way of assuming power over the group and men over women. The discussion went on to the importance but lack of status many felt in their current social, professional, and personal lives.

Theoretically, group analysis occurs within a structured time, space and purpose. Ideally, 90 minutes in the same room each week. However, where groups are held outside a fixed site, external forces frequently sabotage this, often 'the management'.

The doctors' group was a fixed monthly group for senior doctors in a nationally renowned hospital. The group had been brought together as the team they worked with was called to account for a rise in bullying accusations between doctors, nurses, and managers. I, as the group leader, had to accept that whilst the core group members remained the same, others would come and go depending on call commitments, holidays, and the demands of their busy jobs. Each month, the room in which the group was held was different. One month, the group room was in the head of Human Resources – bringing about banter as to whether the room was bugged and bringing out discussions about fear, hate and control. Another month, the group room was in the middle of the chief executive area – a glass room which, whilst not being overheard, could be observed throughout the session.

Leading (facilitating) groups for doctors requires an acceptance of looser boundaries – between group members and between the facilitator (if the facilitator is also a doctor). In most therapeutic groups, other than work reflective practice groups (where members have a pre-existing professional relationship), group members try to avoid obvious personal and professional boundary issues. However, even though this is difficult as group members might start as strangers, it is not uncommon for doctors to rotate to hospital training posts where another group member works. This requires discussion and "rules" around accidental meetings. Equally, such is the world of medicine, where there are usually only two to three degrees of separation between outwardly apparent strangers; many group members might know of or have had acquaintance with another group member or their significant others (relationship partner, work partner, trainers, consultant and so on).

Boundary transgressions were common in all the groups I led. They brought drinks in, came late, or left early, even drank alcohol before groups, took calls or answered bleeps, talked 'shop' and discussed medical issues.

This could be understood as *'normal'* acting out or, perhaps, the unconscious desire not to become a patient, not to become part of a therapy group and move across the divide.

Boundaries convey the creation of a space or a point where things change and where 'I' becomes 'We' and define the 'they' outside the boundary. It is where rules, behaviours, rituals, and norms come into play. A boundary defines how things are done differently – the point in the group where the doctors become patients. The person becomes a patient when they enter the consulting room. But such is the resistance for doctors to do this that it is acted out in their boundary transgressions – testing the facilitator. Boundaries imply belonging. Not surprisingly, belonging was an overwhelming theme of all the groups.

By becoming unwell, doctors in the groups felt they no longer belonged to "medicine" and that they had let the profession down and were excluded from it. Whilst this might be understood (partly) by the doctors in the suspended doctors' group, it was felt even by doctors still in total employment. For doctors, the therapy groups helped address the loneliness of being out of work and improve group cohesion. They provided a safe base to 'open up' without the stultification of discourse and personality growth that theorists might predict.

For example, Peter is a group member in a year-long group. He was a doctor who had a drug addiction – having abused cocaine, cannabis, and alcohol for many years. Currently suspended by the Regulator, he relied on savings and his parents to live. He would often leave the circle and patrol the outside or, more commonly, push his chair back to be outside the circle. When challenged by the group, and over time, what emerged was his immense sense of shame and isolation. Not only was he a sick doctor, but his illness was related to illegal and shameful activity, and he felt excluded from all his medical colleagues, even those in the group.

Yalom writes of universality and a sense of belonging as therapeutic factors in group analysis.[94] If groups of primary belonging are destroyed, then groups of secondary belonging become more significant, mainly were belonging to a group is necessary to sustain a stable sense of self, which is the case for most of the human race. The group of primary belonging for doctors is their work (medicine), which encapsulates their sense of self. Once this has been destroyed (for some doctors, this can be total – for example, suspended doctors are not permitted to set foot inside their hospital or talk to anyone from work during their period of suspension), groups of secondary belonging, the therapy group, become crucial. These groups provide the transitional space, allowing them to assimilate their differences and understand their similarities and for translucent connections to be (re)made that allow for belonging, identity and healing.

In the therapy group, united through their profession, doctors could talk to each other with powerful authenticity without the need to explain or feel (implicitly or explicitly) attacked. The doctors relished rather than rejected the idea of being part of a doctor-only group, and over time, other patients have presented specifically requesting group therapy. Members disclosed sensitive problems, for example, sexuality, suicide attempts, issues with drugs and past childhood abuse. The vulnerability some feared in this unfamiliar setting was counteracted by the sense of safety that 'we're all in the same boat'. I believe anchoring the group in one primary dimension allowed them to appreciate their 'self' in the safety of encounters with 'sameness', and throughout the group life, the members grew psychologically through this experience and learned to be patient.

The group members came late, fiddled with their mobile phones, and left the group mid-session, coming back without comment. They talked between themselves and not to the group. On a scorching day, one doctor kept his coat on in a sweltering room. He looked for all the world like a distressed, battered and hurt child. I reflected on this to him. On another occasion, a doctor had to leave the session to take an urgent call – this was allowed. He returned and somewhat dismissively told the group that a baby he had been looking after had finally died after a painful and long terminal illness. At this point, he tucked his legs under his chin and stared out the window. Another doctor in the room commented that she had been at a failed resuscitation the previous day for an 11-year-old child with a severe respiratory disorder. She, too, stared out into nothingness. Someone made a joke about the temperature in the room being too stiflingly hot as the central heating was on despite it being a scorching day. Silence followed. I talked about the oppressive feeling in the room, which felt like pain. Deeply felt emotional pain, commenting that in the space of 2 minutes, immense pain had entered the room with the deaths of these patients. I wondered where these doctors took their pain. These doctors were the lightning rod for the pain in the hospital – and, given their status, had nowhere to take it. The hospital had split their painful aspects – the death of children and located it into these doctors who had to carry the burden for themselves.

Of course, wearing outside clothes inside might be innocently assumed to be because the group member was cold, but given the ambient temperature, this was unlikely. It is more likely to represent a fear of the group, a fear of exposure, especially vulnerability and a wish to be ready to leave at any moment. This resonated with a recurrent theme in all the groups, especially at the start, which was the doctor's deep regret of becoming a doctor in the first place.

Doctor-only groups might perpetuate the perceived elitism of professionals. However, for doctors needing treatment (for mental health and addiction problems), the evidence suggests that homogenous groups are more beneficial for restoring health due to the process of the group function and *not* due to pandering to professional arrogance. Foulkes ran soldier-only groups, not just for practical reasons (they were inpatients at Northfields) but also from his belief that they had special needs, requiring their homogenous group to address. The same logic applies to doctors with unique problems and a set of deeply constructed barriers to getting effective treatment. Mixing junior- (training grade) and senior-level doctors has been difficult, probably much to do with the power relationships endemic in medicine. Maintaining boundaries needed addressing, as inevitably, some doctors found themselves working in the same hospital, which required discussion and *'rules'* around accidental meetings. There were also issues with me, their conductor. As a doctor, group members view me with idealisation and defer to me for solutions to many professional difficulties. This, however, allowed for a discussion as to why intelligent individuals found it difficult to negotiate their answers and were so powerless when faced with personal (rather than clinical) pressures. This is likely linked to the infantilisation of doctors within a hierarchical profession and unrelenting pressures to be seen as beyond reproach. I am also acutely aware that I represent the medical world from which some had recently been painfully ejected.

Despite initial reluctance, doctors are good at using groups to effect therapeutic change and have excellent outcomes once engaged. Given the shadow side of medicine, where shameful projections are thrown at doctors who express vulnerability, group members often expressed anxiety about being humiliated or judged by colleagues in the group setting during the assessment stages. These fears were always allayed once members identified with their shared struggles. The groups have successfully broken the isolation doctors feel at all medical levels or specialities, normalising our most basic human need for support.

A PERSONAL TALE

Caroline Walker
Psychiatrist and Therapist

Hello, my name is Caroline Walker, also known as *The Joyful Doctor*. I am a psychiatrist and therapist by background, and I have experienced mental health problems, including bipolar affective disorder, addictions, PTSD and an eating disorder. These struggles and the help I received from them over the years led me to specialise full-time in the well-being of doctors. I am passionate about reducing stigma for those affected by mental health problems and role-modelling that it is okay to struggle with your mental health as a healthcare professional.

When I first hit the wards as a junior doctor, I quickly discovered how hard being a doctor is. Everywhere I looked, people were in need, and I felt responsible. I faced people's frustration, disappointment, despair, shock, frailty and pain – which often reflected my own, more hidden but equally intense suffering. Fear and uncertainty were my constant shadows. I couldn't keep up with the never-ending bleeps, the endless to-do list and my internal sense of not being good enough. Everyone else around me seemed to know what they were doing, and I didn't.

As my clinical years continued, I found myself woefully unqualified and inexperienced for the vast array of other roles expected of me – manager, supervisor, teacher, leader, advocate and often enemy. Many of the environments and cultures I worked in were toxic and problematic. There was relentless pressure to perform, with unpredictable and inadequate avenues of praise and support. There was too much to do and insufficient time or resources.

As a doctor, I often found a mismatch between what I *wanted* to do and what I *could* do. I tried to care but couldn't keep watching at the rate and intensity required by the job. I tried to listen but couldn't keep hearing the same thing without zoning out or screaming inside. I tried to heal but would find myself repeatedly impotent in the face of overwhelming disease and mortality. Too often, I would find myself paralysed by my anxiety, indecision, or belief that some other doctor would most likely do this better than I could. This prolonged exposure to traumatic and challenging experiences was physically, emotionally and spiritually draining.

Luckily, it wasn't all bleak. There were times when I loved my work and was able to lead a relatively healthy, happy, and balanced life. Even when I struggled, there were often just enough good bits to keep me going. The grateful relative at five in the morning when I was on my last legs and thinking of quitting.

The patient pulled around at the last moment when all hope seemed lost. The child was born at the end of a difficult shift that made their parents' faces (and mine) explode with love. Much like drinking for a functioning alcoholic, there was often just enough good stuff to keep me returning for more despite the harmful consequences.

Addiction is an apt metaphor to use for working in medicine. As doctors, we often feel compelled to keep doing our work even though it brings us pain. We constantly search for that same 'hit' we used to get from it. Our work takes on greater salience over time, holding a growing prominence in our lives – leaving our health, hobbies, and relationships in their wake. In denial, we passionately defend the medical way of working to its critics, saying that *'they don't understand'*. We start to fantasise about a more leisurely life without it, only to find ourselves paralysed with fear at the thought of letting it go. We make multiple attempts to reduce medicine's hold on us, perhaps successfully for a while, before inevitably ending up back under the mercy of its tightening grip.

Like many addictions, we can find ourselves cycling from pre-contemplation (*'maybe I should think about doing something else'*) through to action (searching for alternative careers on the internet) back to relapse (*'I'll just stick with it for six more months'*). Also, like an addiction, some of us require total abstinence to recover, for whom it becomes essential to leave medicine entirely for a while. Some of us can learn to practice 'controlled medicine' or 'medicine in moderation', know how to manage it and recognise the signs when things are slipping.

The good news is, like any addiction, we can get better and stay better over time. We can learn to live with medicine, even enjoy it again, or move on from treatment with love and gratitude for what it has given us. How do we do this? The answer is **with the help of others**. In my experience, the one thing that has consistently united those recovering from addiction is not the cravings, the tolerance, the fear of relapse – it is the fact that they didn't get better on their own. They recovered by connecting with others, usually some combination of other recovering people with an addiction and professional support. And so, it must be with struggling doctors and healthcare professionals. We need to connect with other doctors and healthcare professionals who have worked – to realise that we are unwell, to accept that we need help and to stay well when we do get better.

When the medical profession heals itself this way, the potential implications for our patients and society are immeasurable and profound. Whether they stay working in medicine or not, each doctor and healthcare professional will touch thousands and thousands of lives over their lifetime. Each interaction is a potentially life-changing moment for both parties and beyond – a chance to learn, grow and heal. We owe it to our patients, to society and to the world to look after ourselves as well as we look after others. We must show ourselves the same compassion that we so willingly show others. It starts with being kind to me and you being kind to you, and then we can all be kind to each other.

19

Self-care

The current healthcare climate is difficult to work in. As such, creating a culture of increased self-awareness and care and a supportive environment where mental health issues can be safely raised will be essential to any doctor's work. Developing resources to maintain one's well-being will be vital.

TEA & EMPATHY

Caroline Walker
Ashley Birtles for 'Tea & Empathy'

In February 2016, Rose, a junior doctor, sadly took her own life amidst a junior doctor contract dispute in the UK. The conflict had caused a bitter and damaging narrative to develop amongst doctors at all stages of their careers, and it had taken its toll on many of us. However, amongst the hurt, anger and fear, there was a growing sense of something positive – a sense of *connection*. A generation of doctors who had hitherto felt disconnected and alone in their experiences was taking to social media in their droves to complain, to dispute, but primarily to feel heard.

When Rose went missing, a fellow junior doctor reached out across the internet to say, *'Please get in touch, it will be ok, we're here to help'*. She invited colleagues across the country to respond with the phrase *'Tea & Empathy'* if they wanted to support their struggling colleagues. She expected a handful to respond; over a thousand names appeared practically overnight. Doctors up and down the country, and indeed across the world, came together to say, *'You are not alone; I am here for you'*.

And so, Tea & Empathy (T&E) was born, a Facebook-based movement which has grown ever since, the start of a wave of human kindness and connection across the NHS and healthcare systems farther afield.

If you'd like to join T&E or benefit by reading some of the amazing posts and comments generated on it, please go to Facebook and search for 'Tea & Empathy

DOI: 10.1201/9781003391500-19

(PUBLIC GROUP)' or put this link into your browser: *https://www.facebook.com/groups/1215686978446877.*

Members come from several different healthcare professions all over the country and internationally.

DEALING WITH STRESS

Matteo Bernardotto
CBT Therapist, Practitioner Health

As this handbook has discussed, medicine has unique challenges and stressors. These include long working hours, shift work patterns, understaffing and the need for more resources. The nature of the job and the resulting feelings of isolation and lack of control are significant contributors to stress. This stress can then negatively impact healthy habits such as physical activity, sleep and eating.

In such a complex and demanding environment, healthcare professionals must prioritise self-care and learn tools to promote well-being. This may involve engaging in physical exercise, getting adequate sleep and maintaining a healthy diet. These practical strategies can serve as essential cornerstones for improving the health and well-being of healthcare professionals.

The principles of self-care are for both the carer and the cared for. While there is an evidence base for some of the practical aspects discussed, it must be acknowledged that the journey of self-care is a deeply personal endeavour, a journey where there will be much trial and error in finding techniques for ensuring that one maintains a sense of integrity in the face of pain and suffering, the face of adversity in the working environment and the looming fear from medical culture.

The first step in the framework for self-care is to acknowledge and accept that self-care is necessary for overall well-being and resilience. This involves recognising the importance of physical, emotional and mental health and prioritising self-care. Individuals should also strive to cultivate self-awareness and practice self-compassion, recognising that they are not immune to the stressors and challenges of their profession.

The second is identifying and understanding personal stressors, including those related to the medical profession. This may involve reflecting on work-related challenges and identifying sources of stress and burnout.

The third is to develop a self-care plan that addresses these stressors and incorporates practices that promote well-being, such as exercise, healthy eating, mindfulness and social connection. It is essential to set realistic goals and prioritise self-care activities that are sustainable and enjoyable. Otherwise, we set ourselves up to fail.

The fourth is to assess and adjust the self-care plan as needed regularly. This involves checking in with oneself and reflecting on what is working well and what may need to be modified.

The fifth and final step is to seek support from others when needed. This may involve connecting with colleagues, friends or family members for emotional support or seeking professional help from a therapist or counsellor. It is not selfish to prioritise their well-being; self-care is not just a one-time event or activity but a continuous and intentional process. It is also essential for practitioners to set boundaries in their personal and professional lives and to practice saying 'no' when necessary. By acknowledging and addressing the challenges of their profession and prioritising their well-being, practitioners can better sustainably serve their patients and communities.

Overall, the framework for self-care is a dynamic and ongoing process that requires self-reflection, self-awareness and a commitment to personal well-being. By prioritising self-care, medical practitioners can enhance their ability to cope with stress, promote resilience and ultimately provide better patient care and remain enthused with their job as carers.

The main messages to take away are as follows:

- Being responsible for others requires being responsible for oneself.

- Self-care is a personal journey with trial and error. It offers principles to help clinicians maintain integrity in facing challenges such as pain, suffering, adversity and fear of medical culture.

- True resilience is an understanding of the power of choice.

- Our choices in difficult situations can transform our sense of self-compassion into compassionate leadership.

- Still, we must first acknowledge and overcome the conceptual flaws that prevent us from making wise choices.

EXERCISE

It is a generally accepted fact, supported by a wealth of evidence, that an active and healthy lifestyle is essential for health and well-being, both physical and mental.[95] Overall, exercise protects against symptoms of depression, reduces symptoms of anxiety and poor sleep, as well as feelings of distress and fatigue, and enhances well-being.[96]

However, sedentary behaviour has increased dramatically over the last decades, with two-thirds of the adult UK population currently classified as inactive. Needs to meet the recommended 150 minutes of moderate physical activity each week. Doctors are not immune to this trend[97] and are therefore at risk of missing out on the benefits of exercise – biological, physical and psycho-social. Low mood and stress appear to be the most significant barriers to exercising, as a perceived lack of support and confidence. In particular, patients with severe depression struggle to engage in physical activity due to low energy and lack of motivation, highlighting the importance of psychological approaches to improve confidence, inspiration and anxiety.[98]

In a complex and demanding environment, healthcare professionals need to master the art of self-care and learn the tools to foster well-being and reduce stress. Engaging in exercise (of any form!), facilitating a good night's sleep, and eating healthily are some of the main practical cornerstones to improving the health and well-being of healthcare professionals.

NUTRITION

Although a healthy and balanced diet is a well-accepted cornerstone of physical and mental well-being, healthcare professionals, particularly shift workers, tend to have worse dietary habits than those working regular hours in the daytime. This may be due to cultural and behavioural factors. For instance, healthcare professionals may feel they have enough knowledge to improve their health and diet without seeking outside help. Work patterns themselves, especially night shifts, may also alter eating habits. Shift workers often show a mismatch in their daily routines and meals compared with those of family or friends.[99]

From a biological viewpoint, nocturnal eating during a night shift has been shown to cause intestinal motility disturbances affecting digestion, absorption and metabolism of nutrients. In fact, at night, the body is programmed to be in a fasting or catabolic state, where glucose from endogenous glycogen stores is released predominantly to fuel brain function at the expense of peripheral tissues, which, therefore, show increased insulin resistance.[99] These night-time changes are thought to be the reason for the higher rate of impaired glucose tolerance observed in shift workers.[100]

Although it appears intuitive to recommend a healthy and balanced diet to all healthcare and shift workers, there is still much we need to understand about non-conforming nutrition patterns. For instance, whether shift workers should eat during the night shift is still being determined. Nonetheless, the table in Box 19.1 shows provisional dietary guidelines for shift workers that encourage healthy eating.[99]

Healthcare professionals work in demanding environments that test physical and mental resilience. This can harm well-being and lead to unhealthy lifestyles, with sedentary activities, poor sleep and unhealthy diet as standard features. This is especially true for those working night shifts and antisocial long hours. Evidence suggests that self-care is invaluable to healthcare professionals, provided they are well-informed and set achievable goals. The beneficial effects of physical activity, good sleep and a healthy diet require personal effort and commitment. Still, they are a safe and effective way to contain and manage the stress and difficulties that define working in the healthcare sector. Whether the goal is to maintain health and well-being or prevent mental and physical illness, regular exercise, good sleep and a balanced diet provide reliable tools for good health and a better quality of life.

BOX 19.1: Sleep hygiene

SHIFT WORK AND NIGHT SHIFT EATING RECOMMENDATIONS

Eat *breakfast before day sleep* to avoid waking due to hunger.

Follow a *normal day and night pattern of food intake* as much as possible.

Divide the day into *three satiating meals over 24 hours*, amounting to 20%–35% energy intake each. The higher the energy needs, the more frequent the eating should be.

Avoid high-energy convenience foods and high-carbohydrate foods during the shift. Instead, choose vegetable soups, salads, fruit salads, yoghurt, wholegrain sandwiches, cheese, cottage cheese (topped with slices of fruits), boiled eggs, nuts and green tea (promoting antioxidant activity). However, this may seem unpalatable to some.

Schedule *adequate sleep and meal preparation* time between shifts.

Avoid sugar-rich products like white bread, soft drinks, bakery items, sweets and non-fibre carbohydrate foods (high glycaemic load).

SLEEP

Sleep is an essential component of the trinity for body discipline: Diet, exercise and sleep. While shift patterns may make exercise challenging, they should still be incorporated into daily routines whenever possible. For example, a 20-minute run before or after a shift could be substituted for a couple of stops on the underground or bus, converting travel time into productive exercise. Factors which stop sleep and why can be summarised in Table 19.1.

Before seeking external interventions for sleep, it is essential to ensure that sleep hygiene is the best before any such intervention, see:

- *https://newsinhealth.nih.gov/2021/04/good-sleep-good-health*

Table 19.1 Improving sleep quality

Tips to improve sleep

Advice	Explanation
Sleep schedule – Set alarm for bedtime and for wake-up time, even on weekends	Changes in sleep patterns disrupt ability to sleep; therefore, sleeping later at weekends due to lack of sleep makes it harder to wake up for Monday morning
Exercise – 30 minutes per day if possible but not 2–3 hours before going to bed	Body temperature may remain raised for a couple of hours after exercise
Avoid caffeine and nicotine	Stimulants disrupt the sleep generation system and may lead to light sleeping only
Avoid alcohol especially before bed	Takes away REM sleep, waking during night
Avoid large consumptions of food and drink at night	Indigestion and urge to urinate at night
If possible, avoid drugs that delay or disrupt sleep	Many cardiovascular drugs can disrupt sleep patterns, as well as some asthma medications and over-the-counter pills
No naps after 3 pm	Reduces ability to sleep at night
Relax before bedtime	Leave time for relaxing activities such as reading or listening to music
Hot bath before bed	Allows for drop in core body temperature after bath and prior to bed
Bedroom environment – dark, cool, devoid of gadgets, turn clocks away from you	Rid the bedroom of any distracting external stimuli
Sunlight – bright lights in morning and/or at least 30 minutes outside in natural sunlight, dim lights before bed	Important for regulating sleep patterns
Bed is for sleep – do not lie in bed awake for more than 20 minutes	Anxiety over sleep hinders ability to sleep

20

And finally

Hopefully, this book has provided the reader with information about identifying, managing and caring for a doctor with a mental illness. What is important is staying well – that those who care for the most vulnerable are themselves attended to.

THE 'RESTORED HEALER'

Sarinda's story continued:

My parents rushed me to an accident and emergency. From there, it was established that I had no insight and was enough of a danger to myself. My two weeks as an inpatient in an adult mental health unit were eye-opening. Far from being a negative experience, I felt loved, cared for and understood. Perhaps the best therapy – and maybe because I could not rid myself of my metaphorical white coat – was engaging with and helping other patients. It is surreal to look into the eyes of another man who has sought death's embrace. Through my blurred, tear-filled vision, I could see his tears too. I was not alone. Spending time with my fellow patients and fellow humans and understanding their suffering made me feel I should live. As with Sisyphus – hell gave me meaning. A tiny flower of care was blossoming in my mind once more. I wanted to help my fellow depressed and psychotic inpatients. I would sit with them, eat with them and enjoy their presence. I shared many a heart-wrenching moment with them. The day of discharge was quite challenging, for I was brought to tears hugging my fellow patients on leaving. It was time for my distressed brothers to reunite with the outside world again.

A second life. Having died once already inside, I was determined to use what energy I had left for a higher purpose. The moment I connected with a stranger over the shared thought of death was when I vowed to do my best to prevent others from reaching this point. I wanted to make reparations with all my loved ones and closest friends. I wanted to start a new path to prevent doctors from reaching the end of suicide. I am still alive because I was caught; no doctor should go through that. Not a human who dedicates their life to caring for others.

 DOI: 10.1201/9781003391500-20

The part of me that remains is healed. It is stronger. It has replaced despair with hope. It is filled with love. But the fear of death is forever gone. A new perspective and time away allowed for reflection. How much did I break myself? How did the system break me? Where was the support? How toxic and corrupt is the healthcare culture? Who does care for us, doctors? How long have all these issues been around? Was this all my fault? There are opportunities where responsibility has been abdicated. Ongoing rhetoric of talking without action. Noise without substance. I want to change this. I want to change a system that is contributing to the deaths of doctors. I want to stop a system from killing us.

As for the part of me that is dead, its spectra mean something to me. All that suffering was for something: It has given me the courage to meet any obstacle. I engaged with NHS Practitioner Health for support through recovery, where I heard the magic words from my treating clinician, 'you do not have to be a doctor'.

I applied and prepared for interviews to London hospitals' health and well-being agenda. Slides of numbers and slides of stats. The NHS People Plan. Equality, diversity and inclusion. I found the irony not only hilarious but deeply insulting to the dead doctors before me when the first question I was asked at an interview for a health and well-being lead was: 'What is a return on investment?' This was when I knew I would not get the job because I would have to commit myself to breaking my values, again, to be forced to create meaningless interventions that served a business in cutting costs and presenting a label to say that they were helping us. I was humbled to hear back from the leadership of NHS Practitioner Health, who kindly put me in touch with Clare Gerada to work on this handbook. What an honour and what a privilege. Finally, I have an organisation to work with, where I feel valued by an understanding mentor, where I can manage myself and where I can make valid contributions with superb feedback.

Following the Wounded Healer Conference, I was thrilled and hopeful, surrounded by outstanding individuals dedicating their lives to helping other healthcare professionals. To be a part of this work is humbling, but a work I want to do justice. I will research and find the wisdom to pass on to others. I will learn from those who are far more experienced than I am. I will aid to the best of my abilities to help doctors in distress. My lived experience has provided insight into the fall to the abyss, and I will also apply any wisdom gained from now to myself so that I can one day be of better service to others. A long, hard road ahead, but these obstacles are the way forward. There is always hope.

References

1. Gerada, C. *Beneath the white coat: doctors, their minds and mental health* (Routledge, 2021).
2. Brooks, S. K., Gerada, C. & Chalder, T. Review of literature on the mental health of doctors: are specialist services needed? *J. Ment Health* **20**, 146–156 (2011). doi:10.3109/09638237.2010.541300.
3. Crawshaw, R. *et al.* An epidemic of suicide among physicians on probation. *JAMA* **243**, 1915–1917 (1980).
4. Imo, U. O. Burnout and psychiatric morbidity among doctors in the UK: a systematic literature review of prevalence and associated factors. *BJPsych Bull.* **41**, 197–204 (2017).
5. Cocker, F. & Joss, N. Compassion fatigue among healthcare, emergency and community service workers: a systematic review. *Int. J. Environ. Res. Public Health* **13**, 618 (2016).
6. Mutambudzi, M. *et al.* Occupation and risk of severe COVID-19: prospective cohort study of 120 075 UK Biobank participants. *Occup. Environ. Med.* **78**, 307–314 (2021).
7. Williamson, V., Lamb, D., Hotopf, M., Raine, R., Stevelink, S., Wessely, S., Docherty, M., Madan, I., Murphy, D. & Greenberg, N. Moral injury and psychological wellbeing in UK healthcare staff. *J. Ment. Health* **32**, 890–899 (2023). doi:10.1080/09638237.2023.2182414.
8. Greenberg, N. *et al.* The mental health of staff working in intensive care during COVID-19. *medRxiv* (2020).11.03.20208322 (2020) doi:10.1101/2020.11.03.20208322.
9. Greenberg, N. & Rafferty, L. Post-traumatic stress disorder in the aftermath of COVID-19 pandemic. *World Psychiatry* **20**, 53–54 (2021).
10. Bennett, J. & O'Donovan, D. Substance misuse among health care workers. *Curr. Opin. Psychiatry* **14**, 195–199 (2001).
11. Brooke, D., Edwards, G. & Andrews, T. Doctors and substance misuse: types of doctors, types of problems. *Addict. Abingdon Engl.* **88**, 655–663 (1993).
12. McAuliffe, W. E. *et al.* Alcohol use and abuse in random samples of physicians and medical students. *Am. J. Public Health* **81**, 177–182 (1991).
13. Milligan, B. Morphine-addicted doctors, the English opium-eater, and embattled medical authority. *Vic. Lit. Cult.* **33**, 541–553 (2005).
14. Myers, T. & Weiss, E. Substance use by internes and residents: an analysis of personal, social and professional differences. *Br. J. Addict.* **82**, 1091–1099 (1987).

15. Boulis, S., Khanduja, P. K., Downey, K. & Friedman, Z. Substance abuse: a national survey of Canadian residency program directors and site chiefs at university-affiliated anesthesia departments. *Can. J. Anaesth. J. Can. Anesth.* **62**, 964–971 (2015).

16. Mayall, R. Substance abuse in anaesthetists. *BJA Educ.* **16**, 236–241 (2016).

17. Kurka, T., Soni, S. & Richardson, D. High rates of recreational drug use in men who have sex with men. *Sex. Transm. Infect.* **91**, 394 (2015).

18. Merlo, L. J., Sutton, J. A., Conwell, T. & Brown, M. E. Psychiatric conditions affecting physicians with disruptive behavior. *Psychiatr. Times* **31** (2014).

19. Rosenstein, A. H. & O'Daniel, M. A survey of the impact of disruptive behaviors and communication defects on patient safety. *Jt. Comm. J. Qual. Patient Saf.* **34**, 464–471 (2008).

20. Hicks, S. & Stavropoulou, C. The effect of healthcare professional disruptive behaviour on patient care: a systematic review. *J. Patient Saf.* **18**, 138–143 (2022). doi:10.1097/PTS.0000000000000805.

21. Zeidan, J. *et al.* Global prevalence of autism: a systematic review update. *Autism Res. Off. J. Int. Soc. Autism Res.* **15**, 778–790 (2022).

22. Ohl, A. *et al.* Predictors of employment status among adults with autism spectrum disorder. *Work Read. Mass.* **56**, 345–355 (2017).

23. Doherty, M., Johnson, M. & Buckley, C. Supporting autistic doctors in primary care: challenging the myths and misconceptions. *Br. J. Gen. Pract. J. R. Coll. Gen. Pract.* **71**, 294–295 (2021).

24. Cassidy, S. Suicidality and self-harm in autism spectrum conditions (2020).

25. Moore, S., Kinnear, M. & Freeman, L. Autistic doctors: overlooked assets to medicine. *Lancet Psychiatry* **7**, 306–307 (2020).

26. Kazda, L., Bell, K., Thomas, R., Sims, R. & Baratt, A. Overdiagnosis of attention-deficit/hyperactivity disorder in children and adolescents. *JAMA Netw. Open* **4**, e215335 (2021). doi:10.1001/jamanetworkopen.2021.5335.

27. Gerada, C. The Wounded Healer: report on the first 10 years of Practitioner Health Service (2018).

28. The bipolar doc: speaker, writer, doctor, teacher. https://thebipolardoc.wordpress.com/blogs/

29. Dome, P., Rihmer, Z. & Gonda, X. Suicide risk in bipolar disorder: a brief review. *Med. Kaunas Lith.* **55**, 403 (2019).

30. Milner, A. J., Maheen, H., Bismark, M. M. & Spittal, M. J. Suicide by health professionals: a retrospective mortality study in Australia, 2001–2012. *Med. J. Aust.* **205**, 260–265 (2016).

31. Hawton, K., Agerbo, E., Simkin, S., Platt, B. & Mellanby, R. J. Risk of suicide in medical and related occupational groups: a national study based on Danish case population-based registers. *J. Affect. Disord.* **134**, 320–326 (2011).

32. Hawton, K. Suicide in doctors while under fitness to practise investigation. *BMJ* **350**, h813 (2015).

33. Elliot, L., Tan, J., Norris, S., & Beyondblue (Organisation). *The mental health of doctors: a systematic literature review* (Beyond Blue, 2010).

34. Gabbard, G. O. The role of compulsiveness in the normal physician. *JAMA* **254**, 2926–2929 (1985).

35. Stienen, M. N. *et al*. Different but similar: personality traits of surgeons and internists-results of a cross-sectional observational study. *BMJ Open* **8**, e021310 (2018).

36. Freud, S. Group psychology and the analysis of the ego. The Standard Edition of the Complete Psychological Works of Sigmund Freud, Volume XVIII (1920–1922): Beyond the Pleasure Principle, Group Psychology and Other Works. 65–144 (1921).

37. Krantz, J. Social defences and twenty-first century organizations. *Br. J. Psychother.* **26**, 192–201 (2010).

38. Frank, E., Nallamothu, B., Zhoa, Z. & Sen, S. Political events and mood among young physicians: a prospective cohort study. *BMJ* **367**, 16322 (2019). doi:10.1136/bmj.l6322.

39. Clarke, R. Zero by Jeremy Hunt review – this is going to hurt. *Guardian* (May 22, 2022).

40. Henderson, M. *et al*. Shame! Self-stigmatisation as an obstacle to sick doctors returning to work: a qualitative study. *BMJ Open* **2**, e001776 (2012).

41. Miles, S. Addressing shame: what role does shame play in the formation of a modern medical professional identity? *Br. J. Psychiatry Bull.* **44**, 1–5 (2020).

42. Rastegar, D. A. Health care becomes an industry. *Ann. Fam. Med.* **2**, 79–83 (2004).

43. Ruggiero, J. S. & Redeker, N. S. Effects of napping on sleepiness and sleep-related performance deficits in night-shift workers: a systematic review. *Biol. Res. Nurs.* **16**, 134–142 (2014).

44. Landrigan, C. P. *et al*. Effect of reducing interns' work hours on serious medical errors in intensive care units. *N. Engl. J. Med.* **351**, 1838–1848 (2004).

45. Hunt, P. A., Denieffe, S. & Gooney, M. Burnout and its relationship to empathy in nursing: a review of the literature. *J. Res. Nurs.* **22**, 7–22 (2017).

46. Pan, K.-Y. *et al*. The mental health impact of the COVID-19 pandemic on people with and without depressive, anxiety, or obsessive-compulsive disorders: a longitudinal study of three Dutch case-control cohorts. *Lancet Psychiatry* **8**, 121–129 (2021).

47. West, M. & Coia, D. *Caring for doctors, Caring for patients* (2019). https://www.gmc-uk.org/-/media/documents/caring-for-doctors-caring-for-patients_pdf-80706341.pdf?la=en&hash=F80FFD44FE517E62DBB28C308400B9D133726450.

48. Oates, A. & Gibbons, R. After a patient dies by suicide: an illustrative case for trainee psychiatrists and trainers. *BJPsych Bull.* **46**, 293–297 (2022).

49. Plunkett, E., Costello, A., Yentis, S. M. & Hawton, K. Suicide in anaesthetists: a systematic review. *Anaesthesia* **76**, 1392–1403 (2021).

50. Shinde, S. *et al*. Guidelines on suicide amongst anaesthetists 2019. *Anaesthesia* **75**, 96–108 (2020).

51. Singh, S. Cultural adjustment and the overseas trainee. *BMJ* **308**, 1169 (1994).

52. Bogle, R. & Lasoye, T. Supporting international medical graduates in the NHS. *The Physician* 6 (2020). https://www.thephysician.uk/supporting-imgs.

53. Gerada, C., Jones, R. & Wessely, A. Young female doctors, mental health, and the NHS working environment. *BMJ* **348**, g1 (2014).

54. Prasad, K., McLoughlin, C., Stillman, M., Poplau, S., Goelz, E., Taylor, S., Nankivil, N., Brown, R., Linzer, M., Cappelucci, K., Barbouche, M. & Sinsky, C. A. Prevalence and correlates of stress and burnout among U.S. healthcare workers during the COVID-19 pandemic: a national cross-sectional survey study. *EClinicalMedicine* 35, 100879 (2021 May 16). doi:10.1016/j.eclinm.2021.100879.

55. Rimmer, A. Nine in 10 female doctors in UK have experienced sexism at work, says BMA. *BMJ* **374**, n2123 (2021).

56. Sontag, S. *Illness as a metaphor* (Collins Publishers, 1988).

57. Moscrop, A. 'Heartsink' patients in general practice: a defining paper, its impact, and psychodynamic potential. *Br. J. Gen. Pract.* **61**, 346–348 (2011).

58. McKall, K. An insider's guide to depression. *BMJ* **323**, 1011–1011 (2001).

59. Tomlinson, J. Using clinical supervision to improve the quality and safety of patient care: a response to Berwick and Francis. *BMC Med. Educ.* **15**, 103 (2015).

60. Wessely, A. "Good addicts, bad patients", Unpublished Social Anthropology Part IIB Dissertation. (Jan 2012).

61. Wessely, A. & Gerada, C. When doctors need treatment: an anthropological approach to why doctors make bad patients. *BMJ* **347**, f6644 (2013).

62. Alexander. General Medical Council. GMC. *Good Medical Practice* (2012).

63. British Medical Association. Ethical responsibilities in treating doctors who are patients (2010).

64. Parsons, T. The sick role and the role of the physician reconsidered. *Milbank Mem. Fund Q. Health Soc.* **53**, 257–278 (1975).

65. Main, T. Some psychodynamics of large groups. In *The large group*, 57–86 (Constable, 1975).

66. Jones, P. *Doctors as patients* (CRC Press, 2022).

67. Bolton, J. M., Gunnell, D. & Turecki, G. Suicide risk assessment and intervention in people with mental illness. *BMJ* **351**, h4978 (2015).

68. Gibbons, R. Eight 'truths' about suicide. *BJPsych Bull.* 1–5 (2003).

69. Schernhammer, E. S., Colditz, G. A. Suicide Rates Among Physicians: A Quantitative and Gender Assessment (Meta-Analysis). *Am. J. Psychait* (2004).

70. Sattar, K., Yusoff, M. S. B., Arifin, W. N., Mohd Yasin, M. A. & Mat Nor, M. Z. A scoping review on the relationship between mental wellbeing and medical professionalism. *Med. Educ. Online* **28**, 2165892 (2023).

71. Bourne, T. *et al.* Doctors' experiences and their perception of the most stressful aspects of complaints processes in the UK: an analysis of qualitative survey data. *BMJ Open* **6**, e011711 (2016).

72. Verhoef, L. M. *et al.* The disciplined healthcare professional: a qualitative interview study on the impact of the disciplinary process and imposed measures in the Netherlands. *BMJ Open* **5**, e009275 (2015).

73. Wallace, J. E., Lemaire, J. B. & Ghali, W. A. Physician wellness: a missing quality indicator. *Lancet Lond. Engl.* **374**, 1714–1721 (2009).

74. Schwartz, H. S. The clockwork or the snakepit: an essay on the meaning of teaching organizational behavior. *Organ. Behav. Teach. Rev.* **11**, 19–26 (1987).

75. West, C. P., Dyrbye, L. N., Erwin, P. J. & Shanafelt, T. D. Interventions to prevent and reduce physician burnout: a systematic review and meta-analysis. *Lancet Lond. Engl.* **388**, 2272–2281 (2016).

76. Kumar, S. Burnout and doctors: prevalence, prevention and intervention. *Healthcare* **4**, 37 (2016). doi:10.3390/healthcare4030037.

77. Panagioti, M. *et al.* Controlled interventions to reduce burnout in physicians: a systematic review and meta-analysis. *JAMA Intern. Med.* **177**, 195–205 (2017).

78. Prochaska, J. O., Velicer, W. F., DiClemente, C. C. & Fava, J. Measuring processes of change: applications to the cessation of smoking. *J. Consult. Clin. Psychol.* **56**, 520–528 (1988).

79. Miller, W. R. & Moyers, T. B. Motivational interviewing and the clinical science of Carl Rogers. *J. Consult. Clin. Psychol.* **85**, 757–766 (2017).

80. Ewing, J. A. Detecting alcoholism. The CAGE questionnaire. *JAMA* **252**, 1905–1907 (1984).

81. McLellan, A. T., Skipper, G. S., Campbell, M. & DuPont, R. L. Five year outcomes in a cohort study of physicians treated for substance use disorders in the United States. *BMJ* **337**, a2038 (2008).

82. Braquehais, M. D., Valero S, Bel, M. J., *et al.* Doctors admitted to a physicians' health program: a comparison of self-referrals versus directed referrals. *BMJ Open* **4**, e005248 (2014). doi:10.1136/bmjopen-2014-005248

83. Gerada, C. *Practitioner Health 10-year report.* 115 (2018). https://www. practitionerhealth.nhs.uk/media/content/files/PHP-report-web%20version %20final%20copy.pdf.

84. Henssler, J. *et al.* Controlled drinking-non-abstinent versus abstinent treatment goals in alcohol use disorder: a systematic review, meta-analysis and meta-regression. *Addict. Abingdon Engl.* **116**, 1973–1987 (2021).

85. Galanter, M., Talbott, D., Gallegos, K. & Rubenstone, E. Combined Alcoholics Anonymous and professional care for addicted physicians. *Am. J. Psychiatry* **147**, 64–68 (1990).

86. Ziegler, P. P. Monitoring impaired physicians: a tool for relapse prevention. *Pa. Med.* **95**, 38–40 (1992).

87. Domino, K. B. *et al.* Risk factors for relapse in health care professionals with substance use disorders. *JAMA* **293**, 1453–1460 (2005).

88. Sathanandan, S., Abrol, E., Aref-Adib, G., Keen, J. & Gerada, C. The UK Practitioner Health programme: 8 year outcomes in doctors with addiction disorders. *Res. Adv. Psychiatry* **6**, 43–49 (2019).

89. Long, M. W., Cassidy, B. A., Sucher, M. & Stoehr, J. D. Prevention of relapse in the recovery of Arizona health care providers. *J. Addict. Dis.* **25**, 65–72 (2006).

90. Xi, X. *et al.* Doctor's presenteeism and its relationship with anxiety and depression: a cross-sectional survey study in China. *BMJ Open* **9**, e028844 (2019).

91. Aronsson, G. & Gustafsson, K. Sickness presenteeism: prevalence, attendance-pressure factors, and an outline of a model for research. *J. Occup. Environ. Med.* **47**, 958–966 (2005).

92. Harrison, J. Doctors' health and fitness to practise: the need for a bespoke model of assessment. *Occup. Med.* **58**, 323–327 (2008).

93. Gerada, C. & Griffiths, F. Groups for the dead. *Group Anal.* **53**, 297–308 (2020).

94. Yalom, I. & Leszcz, M. The therapeutic factors. In *The theory and practice of group psychotherapy*, 1–2 (Basic Books, 2005).

95. Schuch, F. B., Vancampfort, D., Richards, J., Rosenbaum, S., Ward, P. B. & Stubbs, B. Exercise as a treatment for depression: a meta-analysis adjusting for publication bias. *J Psychiatr Res.* **77**, 42–51 (2016 June). doi:10.1016/j. jpsychires.2016.02.023.

96. Jakobsen, M. D. *et al.* Physical exercise at the workplace prevents deterioration of work ability among healthcare workers: cluster randomized controlled trial. *BMC Public Health* **15**, 1174 (2015).

97. Molina Aragonés, J. M., Sánchez San Cirilo, S., Herreros López, M., Vizcarro Sanagustín, D. & López Pérez, C. Prevalencia de actividad física en profesionales de atención primaria de Cataluña [Prevalence of physical activity in primary health care workers of Catalonia]. *Semergen* **43**, 352–357 (2017). doi:10.1016/j.semerg.2016.04.026.

98. Firth, J. *et al.* Motivating factors and barriers towards exercise in severe mental illness: a systematic review and meta-analysis. *Psychol. Med.* **46**, 2869–2881 (2016).

99. Lowden, A., Moreno, C., Holmbäck, U., Lennernäs, M. & Tucker, P. Eating and shift work – effects on habits, metabolism and performance. *Scand. J. Work. Environ. Health* **36**, 150–162 (2010).

100. Van Cauter, E., Polonsky, K. S. & Scheen, A. J. Roles of circadian rhythmicity and sleep in human glucose regulation. *Endocr. Rev.* **18**, 716–738 (1997).

Index

Printed in the United States
by Baker & Taylor Publisher Services